Managing and Coordinating Nursing Care

Managing and Coordinating Nursing Care

Janice Rider Ellis, RN, PhD

Professor of Nursing
Shoreline Community College
Seattle, Washington

Celia Love Hartley, MN, RN

Director of Nursing Education
Shoreline Community College
Seattle, Washington

With 9 contributors

With illustrations by
Margaret Love McAndrew, MAT
Edmonds, Washington

J.B. Lippincott Company   Philadelphia
New York   London   Hagerstown

Acquisitions Editor: Donna Hilton
Coordinating Editorial Assistant: Susan Perry
Project Editor: Melissa McElroy
Indexer: Sandi Schroeder
Design Coordinator: Kathy Kelley-Luedtke
Designer: Susan Blaker
Production Manager: Caren Erlichman
Production Coordinator: Sharon McCarthy
Compositor: Circle Graphics
Printer/Binder: R.R. Donnelley & Sons Company

1   3   5   6   4   2

Library of Congress Cataloging-in-Publication Data

Ellis, Janice Rider.
    Managing and coordinating nursing care / Janice Rider Ellis, Celia Love Hartley : with
9 contributors : illustrators by Margaret Love McAndrews.
        p.   cm.
    Includes bibliographical references and index.
    ISBN 0-397-54798-6
    1. Nursing services–Administration.   2. Nursing–Planning.
I. Hartley, Celia Love.   II. Title.
    [DNLM: 1. Nursing–organization & administration.   2. Patient Care Planning–
organization & administration.   WY 105 E47m]
RT89.E43   1991
362.1'73'068–dc20
DNLM/DLC
for Library of Congress   90-13641
                                                                              CIP

Any procedure or practice described in this book should be applied by the health-care
practitioner under appropriate supervision in accordance with professional standards of care
used with regard to the unique circumstances that apply in each practice situation. Care has
been taken to confirm the accuracy of information presented and to describe generally
accepted practices. However, the authors, editors, and publisher cannot accept any
responsibility for errors or omissions or for any consequences from application of the
information in this book and make no warranty, express or implied, with respect to the
contents of the book.

*Every effort has been made to ensure drug selections and dosages are in accordance with current
recommendations and practice. Because of ongoing research, changes in government regulations and the
constant flow of information on drug therapy, reactions and interactions, the reader is cautioned to
check the package insert for each drug for indications, dosages, warnings and precautions, particularly
if the drug is new or infrequently used.*

Contributors

Mary Ann Anderson MS, RN, CNA
Assistant Professor
Weber State University
Ogden, Utah
Chapter 3   Setting Goals and Objectives

Jeanette Bernhardt MSN, RN
Chairman, Department of Nursing
West Georgia College
Carrollton, Georgia
Chapter 9   Teaching Staff

Ann Boyle Grant PhD, RN
Chairman, Nursing Division
Cuesta College
San Luis Obispo, California
Chapter 2   Developing a Management Style, and
Chapter 13 Using Research

Gerry Hansen EdD, RN
Nursing Program Director/Professor
Weber State College
Ogden, Utah
Chapter 3   Setting Goals and Objectives for Nursing

Barbara Murphy EdD, RN
Director, Council of AD Programs/Council for Nursing Centers;
Consultant, Division of Education and Accreditation
National League for Nursing
New York, New York
Chapter 8   Developing Motivation in Yourself and Others

v

Elizabeth A. Nowlis EdD, RN
Professor of Nursing
Shoreline Community College
Seattle, Washington
Chapter 7   Managing Time Effectively

Thomas J. Smith PhD, RNC
Assistant Professor of Nursing
College of Nursing
University of Southwestern Louisiana
LaFayette, Louisiana
Chapter 6   Decision Making for Patient Care

Martha B. Sparks PhD, RN
Associate Professor of Nursing
Indiana State University
Terre Haute, Indiana
Chapter 12   Becoming An Effective Advocate

Madeline Turkeltaub PhD, RN
Professor and Director, Nursing Program
Montgomery College, Takoma Park Campus
Rockville, Maryland
Chapter 5   Managing Resources Responsibly

Preface

Two factors are primarily responsible for the origination and development of this text. The first, and probably the most important, factor is the deep-seated belief we hold that all nurses are managers. Nurses manage time, care, the patient care environment, resources on any unit, patient teaching and the professional development of themselves and others, and so forth, and so forth. The list can become very lengthy.

Believing this, we are faced with another condition; that is, principles of sound management can be identified, analyzed, critiqued, and researched. Methods can be outlined that result in management being more or less effective. Once we understand what methods are most successful and what factors need to be considered to ensure positive outcomes, we can teach those skills to others.

This brings us to the second major factor responsible for this text—the need for a book that would address management skills from a vary basic, commonsense perspective. As you learned in your basic nursing courses, a need exists when there is a lack of something useful, required, or desirable. When we reviewed the literature available in the area of nursing management, we identified many fine books that discussed the various aspects of management, leadership, and feedback and evaluation. We even found texts that were developed on just one topic related to management skills such as decision making. But we could find none that brought together in one comprehensive text the concepts we felt each new graduate would be expected to know. Thus, we bring to you *Managing and Coordinating Nursing Care*.

This book is designed for use in a course offered at the end, or very close to the end, of a student's program of nursing studies. Its purpose is to introduce students to the basic knowledge and skills related to coordinating and managing patient care that they will be expected to use as they move into the profession of nursing. The book is organized into three major units of study: understanding organizations, facilitating the management process, and developing management skills. Introductions describing the content of each unit can be found preceding that unit in the text.

As you read and become familiar with the content in the book, you will recognize that a number of themes weave in and out of the material presented in the various chapters. For example, you will find a discussion of the process of establishing priorities in the chapter on time management. You must establish priorities effectively to make good use of your time. Similarly, a discussion of priority setting occurs in the chapters on decision making and on developing goals and objectives. Being able to set priorities is a critical step in making sound decisions and in setting meaningful goals. These essential elements of management include, in addition to establishing priorities, concepts related to delegating responsibility; interacting, communicating, and collaborating with others; prompting effective working relationships; using your knowledge of the organization to effect quality patient care; being accountable for the care given; and motivating others to do their best.

We bring to you, then, *Managing and Coordinating Nursing Care.* As with all such projects, the measure of our success will be determined by how useful this material is to you. We encourage your comments, suggestions, and recommendations.

Janice Rider Ellis, RN, PhD
Celia Love Hartley, RN, MN

Acknowledgments

There are many persons we need to acknowledge. First among those must be the individuals who wrote a number of the chapters of this book. You will find their names listed in the contributor section. We are especially grateful to these persons for their sensitivity to tight deadlines, to their positive responses to our comments on first drafts (or second or third), and for their enthusiasm for this project. We express our thanks to our illustrator, Margaret McAndrew, who captured our concepts and made them visual throughout the book. We are also appreciative of the support provided by our respective husbands, Ivan and Gordon, who have had their hand at cooking, cleaning, ironing, or whatever to allow us extra time to develop this text. And our thanks would not be complete if we did not mention the editors of J.B. Lippincott Company for their help. Donna Hilton, in particular, has provided motivation as well as many constructive suggestions as this book has taken shape.

Contents

II
FACILITATING THE MANAGEMENT PROCESS   95

Managing and Coordinating Nursing Care

Understanding Organizations

Before you will be able to function in the role of coordinator and manager of nursing care, you will need a sound understanding of the manner in which organizations function. You must understand organizational structure and hierarchy, communications systems within organizations, and sources of power within the organization. Unit I focuses primarily on understanding the way an organization functions. It explores the various structures that can exist in an organization, examines the many different management styles, talks descriptively of the importance of goals and objectives in any system, and focuses on the significance of power and the types of power that can be found in most organizations. It therefore lays the foundation upon which you will begin to build your skills as a nurse manager and coordinator of care.

Understanding Organizational Structure and Function

1

Objectives

After completing this chapter, you should be able to

1. Examine and describe the structure and relationships of an organization using an organizational chart (include type of structure, span of control, and lines of authority and accountability).
2. Explain the effect on organizational function of a mission statement or a statement of philosophy.
3. Understand the roles of job descriptions and policies and procedures in organizational function.
4. Identify the ways in which the informal organization affects organizational function.
5. Discuss the factors that create the climate in an organization.
6. Identify ways in which a registered nurse would use knowledge of organizational structure and function.

You are surrounded by organizations everywhere. The school you attend, the business for which you work, and your recreational club are all organizations. What differentiates an organization from any other type of group is the presence of a formal structure in which a number of persons have specific responsibilities and are united for some purpose or goal. An organization may be large or small, for profit or nonprofit, efficient or inefficient, but all have certain characteristics based on how they are structured and how they function.

The *structure* of the organization, which is its formal pattern of responsibilities and relationships, underlies its ability to function. This implies that there is a division of labor with different persons having different roles and that there is rank, or a hierarchy, within any organization (Blau & Schoenherr, 1971). Organizational *function* is the way interactions actually occur within the organization. Organizational function is often complex and may be related to characteristics of the employees as well as to the planned structure of the organization itself.

The structure of any organization is designed to allow it to accomplish its purposes. In addition, structure establishes where power in the organization lies and serves to establish a method by which the organization will respond to events and situations. For example, in a hospital the unit nurse manager or the head nurse has responsibilities for day-to-day management of the unit. If an event occurs that is outside of the unit nurse manager's responsibility, the structure of the organization directs the unit nurse manager to the person in the organization who is responsible for handling that type of event.

The structure of an organization also influences individuals within that organization. The position the person fills affects how he or she responds and prescribes certain actions. In return, individuals may have an effect on the organization of which they are a part. Thus, there is always interaction between the individual and the structure of the organization.

As you move into the role of the registered nurse in a health care organization, you will find that you are more successful in accomplishing your goals if you understand how that organization is structured and how it functions. In addition, it will be important for you to understand your relationship with others in the organization in order to meet the expectations for a registered nurse. Who will evaluate me? To whom must I report? To whom can I delegate? Am I responsible for evaluating someone else? To whom do I go with a problem or concern? How do I report errors? These and many other questions are answered by understanding the organization's structure and function.

RELATIONSHIPS WITHIN ORGANIZATIONS

When examining an organization it is important to identify relationships between people and departments. This includes identifying those who have authority or control over others and those who are accountable to specific individuals in authority. *Authority* in an organization is the official ability to control resources and actions. *Accountability* is being responsible to another person for your actions and use of resources. In addition, you will want to consider the number of people or departments one individual supervises and the levels or layers of supervision within an organization.

Chain of Command

The *chain of command* is the path of authority and accountability from one individual at the bottom of the organization to the very top administrative authority. This is also referred to as the *hierarchy* of the organization. For example, a staff nurse reports to the unit nurse manager; the unit nurse manager reports to the nursing supervisor; the nursing supervisor reports to the director of nursing; the director of nursing reports to the hospital

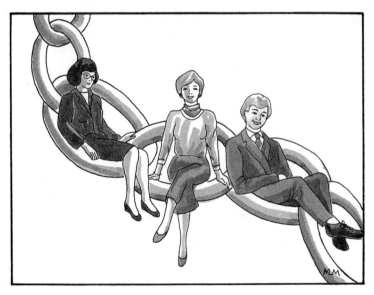

The chain of command is the path of authority and accountability from one individual at the bottom of the organization to the very top administrative authority.

administrator. This is the chain of command for this organization and each person is considered to be on a different level or layer.

Formal communications up and down the organization are directed through the person at the next level. That person is responsible for relaying the message to the next appropriate level. Formal communications are not supposed to skip any levels. Thus, the staff nurse is expected to take concerns to the unit manager and not to the supervisor of the unit manager. If the staff nurse does not feel that there was a satisfactory response at the unit manager level, there is usually some method for the staff nurse to communicate those concerns to the next higher level. Jumping levels in this way usually requires that the individual first exhaust all usual avenues of communication.

Of course, not all communication follows these formal pathways, but this is the design for those communications that deal with conducting the business of the organization. Some organizations adhere closely to these formal lines of communication; others encourage communication outside of these lines if that would be more efficient in accomplishing the desired action. For example, one director of nursing in a community hospital carefully informed all new employees that she maintained an open-door policy. She did not require formal communication lines and, in fact, welcomed communication from individuals throughout the nursing department. She maintained a first-name relationship with all nursing staff and interacted with them in informal ways. In another hospital in that same area, the director of nursing maintained strict formal communication relationships. She expected nurses to make formal appointments through her secretary, expected her secretary to screen individuals regarding the suitability of coming to her with the concern, and systematically redirected concerns back through the formal communication structure. Although the organizational charts of these two hospitals looked similar, the communication pattern was in reality quite different.

Effective function often requires that a manager communicate directly with individuals at many different positions in the organization. Fayol (1949) emphasized that managers on the same level in different departments should build bridges of communication from one to another rather than relying on formal communication going up through one department and down through another. This facilitates problem solving and accomplishing tasks.

Another factor affecting the relationships in an organization is the number of levels between those on the bottom of the organization and those at the very top. The more levels in an organization, the more complex will be its communication patterns. The simplest organization may have only two levels: a person in charge and the workers. In complex organizations there may be a dozen layers of supervisors and managers and administrative personnel above the workers.

Span of Control

In every organization some individuals have more authority and are responsible for directing others. The *span of control* refers to the number of subordinates and different tasks for which a person in authority is responsible. These people or departments are in turn responsible for reporting to the person in authority.

In a narrow span of control the individual will be responsible for only a few people and perhaps one or two task areas. In a broad span of control the individual will be responsible for many people and a wide variety of task areas. Nursing unit managers typically have a narrow span of control, with responsibility for one unit and for a limited number of staff. The highest nursing administrator in one hospital may have a narrow span of control and be responsible only for specific nursing employees. In another hospital the highest nursing administrator may be a vice president for patient services with a broad span of control encompassing diagnostic departments, therapy departments, and outpatient clinics as well as traditional nursing services.

Organizational Charts

An organizational chart is a diagram of the organization that clearly presents its formal structure with persons or departments and their relationships to one another. The organizational chart also provides information on the size of the organization and the chain of command.

Large organizations commonly have an official organizational chart. Small organizations may operate more informally, and an official organizational chart may not be available. If you work in such an organization, drawing a small chart yourself might help you to clarify relationships.

Boxes in an organizational chart may represent individuals in the organization or may indicate entire departments. Solid connecting lines represent communication relationships between individuals or departments. Vertical lines are referred to as lines of authority and accountability. *Lines of authority* represent the responsibility of individuals to supervise others officially. Lines of authority are identified by going downward on the chart. One has authority over those who are lower on the chart and connected by solid lines. *Lines of accountability,* also termed *reporting relationships,* represent a responsibility to report to another person. The same lines that represent authority when moving down the chart represent accountability when moving up the chart. Taken together the vertical lines demonstrate the *chain of command.*

In a hospital, solid lines would connect staff nurses with the unit nurse manager because the unit nurse manager has authority over the staff nurses and the staff nurses are accountable and report to the unit nurse manager.

Horizontal solid lines connect individuals who are at the same level in the organization and have official relationships. These individuals are required to work together for certain objectives in the organization, but none has authority over the others. These equal relationships are depicted by placing individuals on the same level in the organizational chart. In a hospital organizational chart, all the unit nurse managers might be connected by solid horizontal lines to indicate that they have official working relationships but that none has authority over the other. Several might report to the same supervisor.

Dotted lines in organizational charts represent communication relationships in which neither individual has direct authority or accountability to the other and they do not have the same supervisor. For example, the staff development department in a hospital is often connected to other departments by dotted lines. The staff development department has ongoing communication and responsibility toward each nursing unit, but is usually accountable to the nursing administration not the unit. Conversely, the unit works closely with the staff development department but is accountable for actions to the nursing administration office, not to staff development.

Parts of the organization that do not have connecting lines are considered separate units, and formal communication follows the patterns of the lines. Therefore, the official communication between a nursing unit and the housekeeping staff might proceed from the nurses up the solid lines through the nursing department to the point where there are communicating lines between administrators of nursing and administrators of housekeeping. The communication could then move across from the nursing department to the housekeeping department and then down its structure to the appropriate housekeeping person.

TYPES OF ORGANIZATIONAL STRUCTURE

Organizational structures commonly fall into three main patterns: *tall,* or centralized; *flat,* or decentralized; and *matrix.* These patterns also occur in combinations. Each pattern tends to have differing effects on organizational function. You will want to examine the organization for which you work and determine its major pattern and how that pattern affects function in order to work effectively within the organization.

Tall, or Centralized, Structure

A tall organization is so named because a chart of its relationships is tall and narrow (Fig. 1-1). A tall organization is also called centralized because most of the decision-making authority and power is held by a few persons

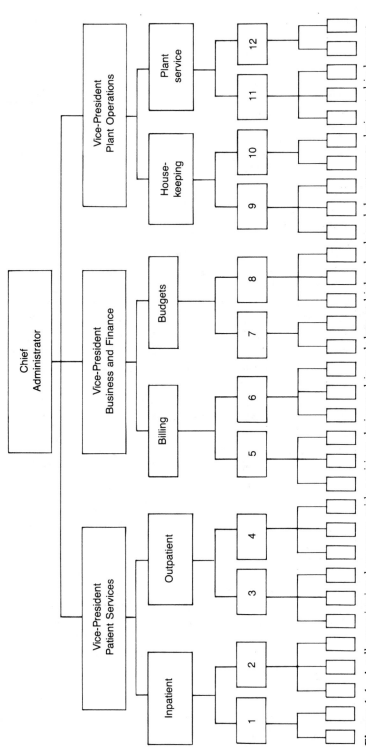

Figure 1-1. A tall organizational structure with positions designated in each box at higher levels and departments designated in boxes at the lower levels.

in "central" positions. In a tall organization each person who has some authority is responsible for only a few subordinates. This is termed a *narrow* span of control. Tall organizations may have many levels, and communication must travel through these many levels.

One advantage of a tall organization is the ability of an individual to be an expert in the narrow area over which he or she is responsible. A tall organization may also make use of many less skilled individuals because the more skilled individuals are placed in positions where they supervise others and procedures are standardized. Because the supervisor has fewer people to supervise (a narrow span of control), there can be close supervision. People at the top of the organization may be spared unnecessary communication if supervisory individuals in intermediate levels screen the communications. Those at the top of a centralized organization have a great deal of control over actions and are the primary decision makers.

These advantages can also become disadvantages. The most skilled individuals may end up doing nothing but supervising while the actual tasks are done by those less capable. Those who are very closely supervised may feel stifled and in extreme cases even mistrusted. Communication is difficult because it must pass through many layers and the person with the authority for decision making may be quite far removed from the actual situation. For the same reason implementation of a decision may be excessively delayed. Some communications never reach the individual who might be able to make a decision for change when that is needed.

Hospitals were traditionally very tall, centralized organizations. A nursing unit might be at the bottom of six or more levels of supervision. Decisions about equipment priorities, staffing patterns, and policies were made at the top levels, and nurses at the lower levels were expected to abide by these decisions. As nurses have moved toward more professional autonomy, they have increasingly found very tall organizational structures restrictive and have sought a variety of ways to have a voice in decision making.

Flat, or Decentralized, Structure

In the flat organization the chart of relationships shows few levels and a broad span of control (Fig. 1-2). In this type of organization, decision making is commonly spread out among many people, and those closest to the situation are given a wide latitude in determining appropriate actions. There cannot be as close supervision when the supervisor is responsible for many people; therefore, the supervisor relies on individuals to make independent decisions. Communication from lower levels to higher levels is easy and direct.

One of the strengths of the decentralized organization is the simplification of communication patterns. With fewer levels there is less

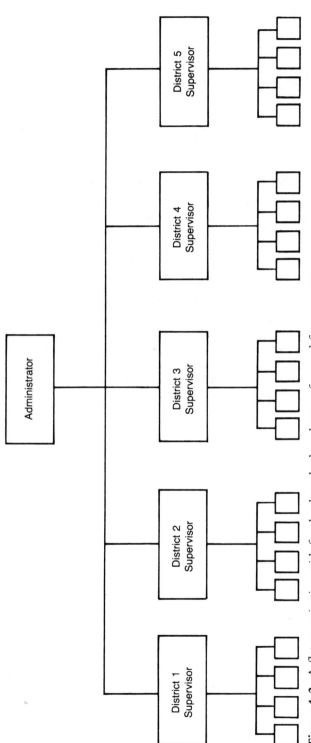

Figure 1-2. A flat organization with few levels and a broad span of control for managers.

chance of messages becoming lost or distorted as they move within the organization. Another asset is the speed with which the organization can respond to problems or new opportunities if decisions do not have to be referred upward through the hierarchy but can be made by those in the situation. Individuals within a decentralized organization have an opportunity to develop their own abilities and autonomy and often see the organization as more humanistic. This leads to greater job satisfaction for the majority of individuals. Many nursing settings are moving toward a more decentralized structure in which nurses directly involved in care have greater autonomy in decision making.

There are also disadvantages to the decentralized pattern. The individual in charge, for example, may have such a broad span of control that the various parts of the organization do not work together as effectively as they might. In addition, the person in charge may find that he or she cannot process all the communication that arrives, or if communication is limited, the supervisor may lack critical information to make decisions at that higher level. The supervisor in a flat organization may lack expertise in the wide variety of operations for which he or she is responsible, thus leading to inappropriate decisions. There is a greater need for ongoing education of individuals within the organization to enable them to make good decisions, and this may be costly. If individuals within the organization are not competent, their inappropriate decisions and actions may do great harm before their lack of ability is identified.

Some health care organizations are moving to a more decentralized model for nursing service. These models take a variety of forms, but common to them is greater decision-making authority by individual nurses. Nurses are sharing in governance through committee structures, primary care for clients, and case management by nurses. Many nurses find this a positive setting in which to practice, because they believe it affords maximum potential for professional growth.

Matrix Structure

A matrix structure may have an underlying structure that is either tall or flat, but its unique characteristic is that a second structure overlies the first, creating two directions for lines of authority, accountability, and communication (Fig. 1-3). This overlying structure represents a special relationship of individuals that is not part of the regular chain of command. Matrix structures are the most recent innovation in health care organizational structure and are often found in very large, multifaceted organizations. Two different situations create matrix structures.

In the first type of matrix, individuals with special expertise serve as resources for a variety of departments. They are not part of the regular chain of command but may still be given some authority over the area in

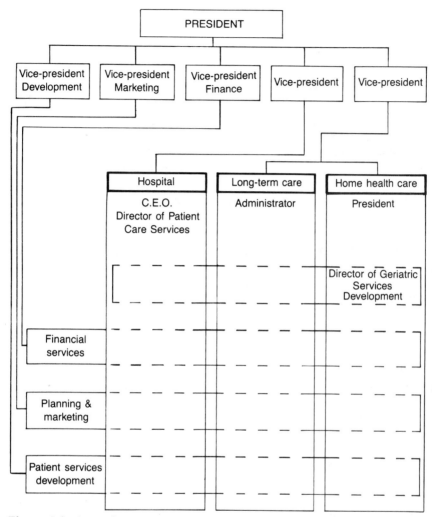

Figure 1-3. A matrix organization with some departments connected by dotted lines representing communication relationships.

which they possess expertise. The advantage of this type of matrix structure is that it provides support from an expert to many segments of an organization.

An example of this type of matrix organization is a corporation that owns many nursing homes. It may employ a nurse who is an expert in gerontological nursing and the reimbursement process for long-term care. He or she may then have responsibility for establishing policies and procedures to maximize reimbursement for all the nursing homes in the group. He or she will also have the authority to see that these policies are carried out. However, this person's position in the organization is in addition to the basic lines of authority and accountability. The nursing director at the individual nursing home is directly accountable to the nursing home administrator for day-to-day operations. The nursing expert will visit, give direction, and perhaps evaluate aspects of nursing. The nursing director will be accountable to this nursing expert as well as to the administrator.

In the second type of matrix, a team approach to problem solving or developing projects is used. A small group with representatives from several departments is appointed to work together. A suitable manager is appointed to lead the group. The members of the team may continue to work part of their time in their base or original department and part of their time with the team.

In the team approach to a matrix, a hospital may decide to develop a health education program for the public. A team composed of persons from nutrition, nursing, physical therapy, and pharmacy may work on this project under the direction of a leader who is a nursing supervisor. Although all members of the team are still responsible to their individual departments, they are also responsible to the team leader for the project.

This dual responsibility and accountability constitute both the advantage and disadvantage of the matrix structure. The assistance and support of an expert can be invaluable when all within the organization work collaboratively. If, however, the administrator and the outside expert have differing goals or priorities, the nursing administrator may be caught between two persons who have authority for directing action. Following the directions of one may cause conflict with the other. This becomes a no-win situation and creates great stress.

A team approach to projects or problems brings together wide expertise and often generates more creative solutions. These team members learn more about each other's concerns, and this may also help with their usual working relationships. However, time allocation between working for the team and working for the base department may become an issue. This is especially true if the base department must operate with a shortage of personnel while the person participates in the team. The team member who will be evaluated by both the team leader and the base department manager may feel a conflict and find it frustrating to be asked to do more than is realistic within the time allowed.

Parallel Organizations

When employees have a collective bargaining organization, that organization parallels but does not usually integrate with the official organization. When nurses are organized for collective bargaining, they may elect officers or representatives to speak for them with the administration.

These representatives may appear on an organizational chart in their role as staff nurses but interact with individuals at higher levels in their role as representatives. Because they speak for many individuals, these elected leaders may have power within the organization. They may participate in bargaining for a contract that outlines wages and working conditions and process any grievances that arise. These leaders will not appear on an organizational chart, but they are very important.

PLANNING FOR ORGANIZATIONAL FUNCTION

Most organizations have written documents governing function within that organization. These statements often take the form of mission and philosophy statements, job descriptions, and policies and procedures.

Mission and Philosophy Statements

A *mission statement* is a broad general goal for an organization that describes its purpose in the community. The mission statement of a small community hospital may indicate that its purpose is to serve the health care needs of the immediate community and provide for care for commonly occurring illnesses and first-line diagnosis. A large university hospital may have a mission statement that encompasses research, teaching, and care for rare or complex problems. These two organizations will establish different priorities for spending, choose different technologies as essential to their missions, and structure their staff in different ways. These mission statements provide the overall umbrella under which all functions of the organization take place. The small community hospital might not encourage individuals to engage in research, and the large university hospital might admit only patients who meet the criteria for research studies under way in certain units. When the budget is prepared, the large research hospital might include an entire department that works with research and statistics. The small hospital might decide not to include a very expensive diagnostic tool. Thus, the mission statement guides planning.

A general *statement of philosophy* is sometimes written in addition to or even in place of a mission statement. When both are present they should be related. The philosophy is typically longer and more detailed. It will reflect the purpose of the organization, will provide a statement of beliefs and values that are basic to its operation, and may include a list of goals or objectives.

Within a hospital a department of nursing often has a philosophy of nursing. This reflects the theory of nursing being used, the values and beliefs regarding nursing in the acute hospital setting, and a list of goals for nursing. A philosophy statement should be used as a basis for determining more specific goals and objectives each year. (See Chapter 3, Establishing and Evaluating Goals for Nursing.)

Job Descriptions

Position or job descriptions also help to define organizational structure and function. *Job descriptions* are written statements describing the responsibilities of each individual or position within the organization. A formal job description never gives a complete description of everything an individual does as part of his or her job, but it should provide the broad general guidelines under which the individual will function. For example, the job description for a nurse in a hospital that has a primary nursing system in place will be quite different from the job description for a nurse in one that has a team nursing system. Even within the same institution, the job description for the nurse in an outpatient clinic will be quite different from that for the nurse in critical care.

Policies and Procedures

Policies and procedures are the official statements of the organization that guide the behavior of individuals. Policies are statements of expected responsibility and the general course of action for a given situation. Procedures are step-by-step guidelines of how one is to do a task. For example, a hospital policy may be, "All emergency surgeries performed on a minor without the written consent of the parent or guardian must be recommended by two surgeons as essential to safeguard life." The procedure for emergency surgery on a minor would then provide the detail of what forms are to be completed and filed, who is responsible for those forms, who in the hospital hierarchy is to be notified, and so forth. These policies and procedures would be written to ensure that all the requirements of the relevant law were met in the situation. Written policies and procedures are required and evaluated by accrediting agencies such as the Joint Commission for the Accreditation of Health Care Organizations (JCAHO).

Hospitals and other health care organizations tend to have many policies and procedures carefully written out in detail. Policies and procedures serve as a legal safeguard for the organization by establishing standards for practice. They may also assist personnel in determining correct practice in an individual situation. The hospital has general policies and procedures that guide the behavior of the entire institution. In addition, the nursing department has policies and procedures specific to its function.

Nursing policies and procedures are most often formulated by committees of nurses working together. In some instances an attorney is consulted to assure that legal requirements are being met. Committee members research the literature and bring together their collective expertise in order to establish the best standard of care. An example of a nursing policy is, "A registered nurse may initiate an intravenous access for a patient without a physician's order when, in the judgment of the nurse, a sudden change in the patient's condition makes the need for intravenous fluids or medications a high probability." Examples of such situations may be provided to assist in the interpretation of the policy. The procedure would then provide specific procedures on starting I.V.'s and the type of solution to be used.

Policies and procedures provide support for good practice and help to ensure consistency and control quality within the organization. However, some nurses may feel constrained by the existence of many policies and procedures because they do not allow for as much individual decision making relative to the unique situation. Moreover, they are difficult to keep current. Health care changes rapidly, and the time necessary to develop good policies and procedures may work against having them reflect the most current information.

Some organizations have relatively few policies and procedures. Instead, these organizations rely on individuals to make decisions in each situation based on their own knowledge and expertise. This provides the broadest possible professional autonomy for the individuals involved and the most flexibility in adapting to the new or unusual situation. It also is the most demanding in terms of the required level of expertise. The individual employee has fewer guidelines and far more responsibility and accountability. The organization itself is more vulnerable to problems created by incorrect decisions, and there is less control over the actions of individual employees.

THE INFORMAL ORGANIZATION

In addition to the formal organizational structure and its function, you will also encounter an informal organizational structure. This will not be drawn out in explicit terms, and the lines of authority and accountability may be blurred and shifting. Nevertheless, it is important and powerful.

Informal organizations arise to meet the needs of the people within an organization. In a very structured organization, the informal organization may provide for ease of relationships and ways to accomplish desired outcomes without using the entire formal structure. In an organization that has a very loose formal structure, the informal organization may provide the additional structure that some people need to function comfortably.

Meeting Social Needs

Social needs are commonly met by the informal organization. Within the informal organization, a person may be viewed more as an individual and a friend than as a worker. Through informal association a person may find a sympathetic ear when he or she is troubled and friends with whom to rejoice when there are joys and successes in life. The informal organization may bring a sense of belonging that is not present in the formal organization.

In some employment settings you will find people celebrating birthdays, planning holiday parties, and creating opportunities for social interaction in other ways. In other employment settings the individuals have independent social relationships that do not include people at work. Some people welcome the opportunity to socialize with those at work; others prefer to keep work life and social life completely independent.

Accomplishing Goals

In addition to its effects on the personal lives of workers, the informal organization may contribute significantly to the success of the organiza-

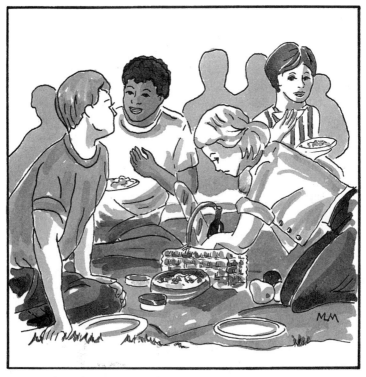

Social needs are commonly met by the informal organization.

tion in meeting its goals. People may assist one another based on their informal relationships, even though the formal structure does not mandate this. For example, on a nursing unit the housekeeping staff may be organizationally quite separate from the nursing staff. An informal working relationship might create cooperation that results in housekeeping people working closely with nurses to make sure that units are promptly cleaned and coordinated with admission needs. Very often these informal relationships are built over time as favors are done in both directions. These relationships rely for their existence on both parties contributing. If one person fails to contribute, the relationship will be lost.

Providing Communication

The informal organization often provides a means of communication and disseminating information that is flexible and personal. Some formal channels are inadequate for the information needs of individuals; thus, the needs are met through the informal organization.

Sometimes an organization may deliberately withhold information from those with less authority. These individuals may want and need some means of obtaining the information that is important to them. The informal organization provides the mechanism. For example, in some businesses, information regarding the budget and whether a profit is being made is a closely guarded secret. An employee who plans to ask for a raise in salary may find this information important. An informal relationship with an employee in the business office may yield the general knowledge that the business is doing well financially, thus allowing the person to negotiate for the raise from a stronger position.

Sometimes the informal organization communicates important information for job performance that the formal organization has not identified. On a nursing unit a new nurse may need to know how nurses share workload when unforeseen events occur. This would not be covered in a formal policy but is very important to effective functioning.

Preserving Values

The informal organization tends to preserve the values of the group. On some nursing units you will find an informal standard regarding participation in continuing education. It is the expectation that everyone will participate and that others will offer whatever support is necessary to make this possible. On another unit, you might not find this same value, nor would you find the corresponding actions to support continuing education efforts by individuals. If the group culture expects conformity to mediocre standards, it undermines efforts of individuals to move toward excellence.

Informal Leaders

Within the informal organization there may be varying levels of status and informal leaders. These informal leaders may wield far more power than their official title or position in the organization would indicate. Some informal leaders are charismatic in their effect on others. Others may be leaders based on specific abilities and actions in job performance. Informal leadership may change based on the situation.

Problems of the Informal Organization

The informal organization may be detrimental to the formal organization as well as a support to it. If the leadership of the informal organization undermines the authority of the formal leader, the result may be lessened effectiveness. Sometimes the informal organization may resist needed change and undermine efforts to achieve new ways of performing. The informal organization may tolerate mediocrity and may even discourage those who would try to demonstrate excellence or ambition. Sometimes the social organization is closed, and new individuals remain outsiders. This may make the work environment unpleasant and create turnover among those who feel they are outsiders. If the social organization expects individuals to invest a lot of time in group activities, the person who does not want to socialize with coworkers may not fit in and therefore may seek employment elsewhere.

A danger of informal communication is that it may also disseminate rumor and inaccurate information. We have all had experiences with "grapevine" messages that create anxiety. Someone has heard that an entire unit will be closed and staff laid off. Everyone is upset. Later this is found to be a false rumor. It is important to be wary of messages that promote extreme views or that are detrimental to relationships and reputations. You should always check the accuracy of informal communications.

ORGANIZATIONAL CLIMATE

Just as the physical climate, hot vs. cold, rainy vs. sunny, affects your ability to carry out certain activities, the psychological climate affects your ability to carry out activities in the organization. The *climate* of an organization refers to the prevailing feelings and values experienced by individuals. The feelings of trust, belonging, esteem, and loyalty are a part of the climate. Values for competence and accomplishment are also part of the climate. The climate is based on the official policies and procedures of the organization, the behavior of supervisors, the informal organization, and the feedback provided within the organization.

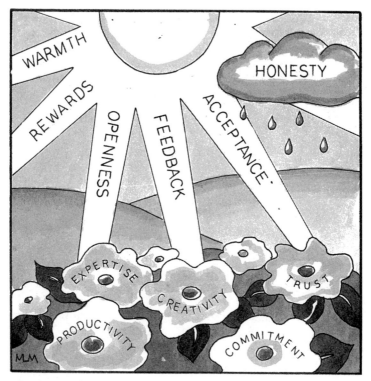

The climate of an organization refers to the prevailing feelings and values experienced by individuals.

The Effect of Policies

Formal policies describe expected behaviors and limit the amount of discretion that an individual is permitted. These policies may be structured on basic philosophies of how people are motivated and respond. In Chapter 8 you will learn more about theories of motivation, but here we will mention two beliefs about motivation that create very different climates.

McGregor (1960a) described some organizations as being operated based on Theory X. The assumptions of Theory X are that people do not like to work, that they are motivated only by material gain, and that without close supervision they will not remain on task. Other organizations he described as based on Theory Y (McGregor, 1960b). Theory Y is based on the assumptions that people find work intrinsically rewarding; are motivated by many factors other than material gain, such as the opportunity for growth and creativity; and can be trusted to do their best.

Still another type of organization, termed Theory Z, was described by William Ouchi (1981). This type of organization operates on the basis of long-term employment, loyalty between employer and employee, and a strong collective value system about maintaining and supporting the organization's goals.

It is clear that policies established with one theory in mind will create a very different psychological climate from policies established with the other in mind. For example, a hospital that operates based on Theory X may set up time clocks in each department and require individuals to punch in and out for breaks and lunch as well as for arrival and departure. This allows for surveillance to assure that no one takes more than the allotted breaks and that a person is paid only for hours worked.

A hospital based on Theory Y may have a very informal system in which nurses submit a signed statement of the specific shifts worked and no attempt is made to monitor breaks, lunches, and so on. The hospital based on Theory Y relies on individuals to monitor themselves and do their job conscientiously.

The nurses in each of the these two organizations will perceive the climate differently in terms of trust in their professionalism. Such policies affect their feelings about the esteem in which they are held and their loyalty to the organization.

Policies may also relate to work expectations, accomplishments, and the level of excellence toward which workers are expected to aspire. If continuing education is supported through payment of fees, education on paid time, and promotion or salary increment for educational accomplishment, the organization is sending a clear message regarding the value placed on education and advancement.

The Effect of Supervisory Behavior

In addition to the formal policies and procedures, the manner in which supervisory personnel carry out these policies and procedures also contributes to climate. The personality of the supervisor and his or her general method of interacting with others has a major effect on the climate in any organization.

The official policy may seem restrictive when it is read, but an individual supervisor may interpret the policy broadly, giving individuals the benefit of latitude in expectations. By word and deed the supervisor may say to the staff, "I trust in your commitment to patient care" and "I value your contribution." Staff members may be supported when they risk failure by trying something new or may be so harshly criticized for failure that they are unwilling to take risks. When the official policy supports continuing education, the immediate supervisor often makes the policy a reality through careful scheduling and consultation with staff. Conversely, the official policy may have little effect if the supervisor does not make the effort to adjust scheduling or otherwise support the individual in attempting to gain more education.

The supervisor does not have to be friends with other employees, but a concerned and friendly approach to interactions makes a difference in the general climate. Some supervisors create an atmosphere of suspicion and fear through their criticism and unwillingness to tolerate less than perfection. Chapter 2 discusses the various management styles in greater detail, and Chapter 11 provides guidelines for giving feedback. As you study them, reflect on the effects these management styles and guidelines would have on the climate of an organization.

The Informal Organization and Climate

The way individuals relate on a personal basis within an organization has a profound effect on the climate. All the factors mentioned when the informal organization was first discussed affect climate. For example, if the informal relationships are based on trust, honesty, and working cooperatively, these feelings will permeate the organization. Some organizations have a high level of competition, but this competition is accompanied by respect for others and a sense of fair play. Consequently, it creates a positive climate. However, if the accepted approach to the job is one of "me first," without concern for the effects of one's actions on others, the climate will be quite different.

Relationships in some organizations are quite formal, with all individuals being addressed by last names and title. In other organizations relationships are informal, with everyone being called by their first name. Neither situation is intrinsically better, but the climate each creates is different.

USING YOUR KNOWLEDGE OF THE ORGANIZATION

There are many ways in which you as a beginning registered nurse can use the information you have gained in this chapter. Here we will discuss a few of them. As you work, additional ways in which you can use this knowledge will become apparent to you.

Identifying Your Own Responsibilities

When you first begin a job, you must learn what your own responsibilities are as quickly as possible. Although these will be reviewed in an orientation program, you cannot expect that you will remember everything that was said during six to eight hours of classes. You can familiarize yourself with the various documents that will assist you as you work. You should know where policy and procedure manuals are kept and what kinds of information are contained in them. Then you can consult them for specific information when the need arises.

You will want to check on your official job description. From there you can check on who will be evaluating you, to whom you are accountable, and from whom you can gain information you need. Some hospitals assign new employees to a preceptor or mentor to fulfill the need for an information source. If your employing agency does not do this, seek out someone who is willing to fulfill this role for you.

Remembering that the informal organization is very powerful will lead you to examine the setting carefully to further your understanding of the values and behaviors that are found in your particular work environment. You will want to observe for the informal leaders and identify how they affect the setting and other employees.

Solving Problems in the Organization

When you encounter a problem in your work setting, you will want to solve it as effectively as possible. One important aspect of this is a review of the organizational structure and function that enables you to determine where to direct your concerns. Should this concern be directed to your immediate supervisor? Should this concern be directed to a specific committee? Should both of these actions be taken? If both are taken, which one is appropriate first? If the problem is not solved, where is the second avenue of action? Is there a role for a collective bargaining representative in this situation?

Each organization has its unique characteristics. In one organization you might find that it is useful to engage the cooperation of a particular informal leader in any proposal for change. You may learn that this person's influence is widespread and can be very effective in either facilitating or blocking change. In another organization a collective bargaining agreement may give power to an elected representative of the staff. In that case you would want to consider whether the issue under consideration is one that relates to the responsibilities of this representative. In many different ways the organization's structure and function will affect your actions.

Changing the Organizational Climate

Organizational climates are not static; they change. Although most changes in organizational climate occur gradually as the people in the organization change and each brings a different approach to the work setting, you can change an organizational climate through deliberative action.

When planning for any kind of change, refer again to the basic nursing process approach you learned early in your nursing program. First, assess the current organizational climate. What is the climate of the work setting? Is this the tone that you would like to see? Clearly state to yourself the problem you see with the climate. Then assess the factors that contribute to it in this particular setting. There will be both negative and positive factors. What actions contribute to this tone? Are there policies and procedures that have an effect on the climate? Is there a particular individual within the organization who is responsible for the climate? Identify as many of the determinants of the organizational climate as you can.

Once you clearly understand the situation as it is and have identified what the problem is, you need to set a clear goal for a new, changed climate. What exactly would you like to see in this new climate? Would you like to see a greater sense of trust? more feeling of autonomy? a stronger support for achieving excellence? Try to set your goal in a realistic way. We would all enjoy a perfect work setting, but that is not going to happen; however, we may be able to improve our work situation.

Once you know where you are and where you want to go, you can begin planning the actions that will get you to your goal. Some of the factors affecting climate may be out of your control, but you may be able to affect others directly. You may change the way you relate to others and begin noting evidence of those aspects you would like to see increased. You may involve others in the change process. If you have identified a problem, others may have identified it also. Such things as policies and procedures may be changed through the prescribed route. This may involve the actions of committees and consultants as well as of those individuals in the specific situation.

SUMMARY

In this chapter we have examined the meaning behind organizational charts in order to help you understand lines of authority and accountability, the concept of span of control, and the effect of the level of a person on his or her role in the organization. The structure of an organization affects the way it functions. An organization's structure may be described as tall (centralized), flat (decentralized), or matrix. Each of these organizational types has strengths and weaknesses.

Formal functioning of an organization is directed through mission and philosophy statements, job descriptions, policies and procedures. These give both overall guidance to employees at every level and detailed guidance for behavior in specific situations.

The informal organization meets social and communication needs of employees. In addition, it may assist with effective attainment of goals and preservation of values within the organization. Informal leaders arise within organizations and are able to influence others. These informal leaders may make an important contribution to the organization's functioning, but they may also be counterproductive. Other problems that may originate within the informal organization include distortions in communication, support for nonproductive behavior, and resistance to accepting new individuals within the social structure.

The organizational climate is the tone that is created by the combination of formal and informal organizational components as well as by the individualized actions of supervisory personnel. Climate is not static but may be affected by many things.

As a beginning nurse there are many ways you can use knowledge of the structure and function of any organization where you are employed. You will need to identify your own responsibilities from the beginning of employment. As time continues there may be problems you will want to help to solve or a climate you wish to change. Your knowledge will be important to you in all these endeavors.

Study Questions/Activities

1. What differentiates an organization from other types of groups?
2. Investigate the organizational chart of the facility where you are currently enrolled for clinical practice.
    a. Would you describe the structure as tall, flat, or matrix?
    b. Are the lines of accountability and authority clear?
    c. To whom would a staff registered nurse on the unit to which you are assigned report?
    d. How would you describe the span of control of the unit nurse manager or head nurse?
    e. What are the main components of the job description for the staff nurse?
3. Investigate the policies and procedures of the health care facility where you have your clinical experience.
    a. Are these policies clear?
    b. What philosophy toward workers do these policies support?
    c. Do these policies and procedures give a wide margin of decision making to individuals or is individual decision making limited?
4. What factors in an organization are affected by the informal organization?
5. Describe the climate of an organization for which you have been employed in terms of the feelings of trust, belonging,

esteem, and loyalty and in relationship to the prevailing values regarding competence and accomplishment.

6. Identify one aspect of the climate you identified earlier that you would like to see changed. Plan strategies that could be used to alter that organizational climate.

REFERENCES

Blau, P.M., & Schoenherr, R.A. (1971). *The structure of an organization.* New York: Basic Books.

Fayol, H. (1949). *General and industrial management.* New York: Pitman.

McGregor, D. (1960a). Theory X: The traditional view of direction and control. In *The human side of enterprise.* New York: McGraw-Hill.

McGregor, D. (1960b). Theory Y: The integration of individual and organizational goals. In *The human side of enterprise.* New York: McGraw-Hill.

Ouchi, William G. (1981). *Theory Z: How American business can meet the Japanese challenge.* Reading, Mass.: Addison-Wesley.

SUGGESTIONS FOR FURTHER READING

Aledina, S., & Funke-Furber, H. (1988). First line managers: Optimizing the span of control. *Journal of Nursing Administration 18f*(5), 34–39.

Boulerice, M. (1989). Management and philosophy statement help set goals and objectives. *Dimensions of Health Services 66*(1), 28–29.

Coeling, H.V.E., & Wilcox, J.R. (1988). Understanding organizational culture: A key to management decision-making. *Journal of Nursing Administration 18*(11), 16–24.

del Bueno, D.J. (1989). Our actions drown out our words: Incongruities between what we practice and what we preach. *RN 52*(8), 100.

Herzberg, F., et al. (1959). *The motivation to work.* New York: Wiley.

McClelland, D., et al. (1953). *The achievement motive.* New York: Appleton-Century-Crofts.

Porter-O'Grady, T. (1987). Shared governance and new organizational models. *Nursing Economics 5*(6), 281–286.

Professionalism of hospital nurses linked to staff structure (1988). *Journal of Nursing Administration 18*(11), 44.

Przestrzelski, D. (1987). Decentralization: Are nurses satisfied? *Journal of Nursing Administration 17*(11), 23–28.

Singleton, E.K., & Nail, F.C. (1988). Nursing leadership: The effects of organizational structure. *Journal of Nursing Administration 18*(10), 10–14.

Strasen, L. (1989). Values and vision in chaotic times. *Journal of Nursing Administration 19*(3), 4–5.

Developing a Management Style

2

Objectives

After completing this chapter, you should be able to

1. *Compare four theories about the nature of leadership.*
2. *Identify three styles of management and the advantages and disadvantages of each.*
3. *Analyze an example of management in terms of its predominant style and its appropriateness to the situation.*
4. *Discuss the role of follower and the characteristics of effective and ineffective followers.*
5. *Develop a plan for beginning to build your own effective management style.*

Nursing students frequently find it difficult to relate to discussions of leadership and management, particularly if they have gone into nursing specifically to work at the bedside, giving direct patient care. You may find at this beginning point in your professional education that thoughts of management and leadership may seem remote from your goals and interests. It is important to understand, however, that all nurses function as leaders and managers, whether they are identified as such by title.

In addition, understanding that you will be both a leader and a follower is critical to the understanding of both roles. At the same time that the staff nurse is serving as a leader and manager in delivering care to patients, the staff nurse also has an important responsibility as a follower. Staff nurses are assisted by supervisors, charge nurses, patient care coordinators, or other leaders formally designated by the institution as managers. It is important for you to understand and be comfortable with the roles of both leader and follower if you are to function effectively as managers in your own spheres of responsibility.

DIFFERENTIATING LEADERSHIP AND MANAGEMENT

Leadership involves the guiding, teaching, and directing of others. "Leadership is the process of influencing the activities of an organized group toward goal setting and goal achievement" (Stogdill, 1950, p. 4). At the top levels of nursing management, the nurse leader may be the Director of Nursing Service, who has overall responsibility for guiding and directing the entire nursing staff and for developing the relationship the nursing department has with the rest of the hospital. At the patient care level of nursing leadership, management involves the coordination of care for a particular patient. The staff nurse works in conjunction with others. He or she delegates responsibilities for particular aspects of the patient's care and coordinates other nonnursing staff to provide for the overall care of the patient.

Management is sometimes confused with leadership, but in fact it is only one component of leadership, which is a much broader role. "Management is the coordination and integration of resources through planning, organizing, directing, and controlling in order to accomplish specific institutional goals and objectives" (Sullivan & Decker, 1988, pp. 209–210). The leadership style a nurse adopts can influence her effectiveness as a manager and is something all nurses, regardless of their position in the institutional hierarchy, should carefully study and develop appropriately.

It is important also to recognize that leadership and management roles are not ones that come easily to many nurses. The reasons for this are multiple and include such things as the public image of nursing, the historical dependence of nursing upon medicine, and the traditional dependence of women upon others. In the public mind, nursing continues to be associated with concern for others, honesty, idealism, and warmth. Nurses are perceived as being less logical, less intelligent, and less extroverted than physicians and as being generally more feminine in orientation (Kaler, Levy, & Shaul, 1989). Traditionally, the exercise of power and authority has been viewed as antithetical to femininity and as more appropriately left to those naturally suited for leadership, namely, men. These views of leadership and authority ignore the fact that increasing numbers of nurses are male and physicians female. More importantly, nurses of both sexes have just as great a capacity and need for the exercise of leadership as do those in other professions.

An additional reason for the reluctance of nurses to see themselves as leaders and managers is that nurses historically have not been prepared to function in these capacities. O'Grady (1989) points out that many nurses are participating in an unparalleled fashion in the management of their practice settings. In organizations implementing a shared governance structure, staff nurses share decision-making authority with the chief nurse administrator; have direct input into budgeting, staffing, and quality-of-life issues; and serve in an official capacity on the governing board. Nurses must understand management as an important part of their responsibilities and undertake to prepare themselves to participate appropriately at all levels.

Outside the acute care hospital setting, the importance of nursing management skills is equally great. In discussing the problem of measuring and predicting the need for nursing care by home health clients, Storfjell (1989) points out that traditional ways of examining this service neglect to factor in the complexity of the task and the need for coordinating the service as a whole. The coordination and direction of complex interactions are management functions. Nurses in community settings require both clinical competency and management skills to deliver appropriate nursing care.

As it becomes evident that all nurses need and use management skills and knowledge, the importance of studying and learning about leadership and management also becomes clear. Just as nurses need the skills of physical assessment and knowledge of pathophysiology, they need the skills and knowledge of management in order to deliver the level of care required by their patients.

In this chapter we will look at various theories about the development of leadership and about the ways in which leaders and followers interact. We will look at three basic types of management and the advantages and disadvantages of each.

We will examine some strategies for evaluating your own leadership style and those of managers you might use as role models. Finally, we will make some suggestions to new graduates on how to begin to develop a responsive management style and how to work collaboratively with both leaders and followers.

THEORIES OF LEADERSHIP

It is helpful in looking at theories of leadership to use an example showing how the various theories would explain the emergence of a leader. For our purposes we will review briefly the history of one very important leader, Florence Nightingale, and then examine how the different theories would explain her leadership.

Nightingale was born in 1820 to wealthy English parents. She was highly educated for her day and especially for her sex, knowing several languages and having studied literature, philosophy, religion, history, political economy, science, and higher mathematics (Donahue, 1985). She became interested in nursing at an early age but was not encouraged by her parents, who felt that it was an inappropriate choice for a lady of her standing, particularly given the situation current in most hospitals of the time. She nonetheless persisted in her goal and proceeded to learn as much as possible about nursing in her travels and studies at Kaiserswerth, Germany, and with the Sisters of Charity at the Maison de la Providence in Paris. During this period she made the acquaintance of individuals who would later be of great assistance to her socially and politically.

This background served to prepare her well for the great challenge presented by the horrors of the Crimean War. When the squalid conditions under which wounded British soldiers were being treated became public knowledge, there was a general outcry for the establishment of an institution of nursing that could provide care similar to that provided by French nurses of the Order of the Sisters of Charity.

One of the influential persons Nightingale had become acquainted with was Sir Sidney Herbert, at that time Secretary of War. Knowing of her commitment to and her knowledge of nursing, he wrote to her, asking her to establish a nursing service to see to the needs of the wounded British soldiers. Rarely has the scope of the charge or the degree of responsibility been greater in any assumption of leadership! After citing the many problems, Sir Sidney wrote to Nightingale:

> My question simply is, Would you listen to the request to go and super-intend the whole thing? You would of course have plenary authority over all the nurses, and I think I could secure you the fullest assistance and co-operation from the medical staff, and you would also have an unlimited power of drawing on the Government for whatever you thought requisite for the success of your mission [Woodham-Smith, 1951, p. 88].

Nightingale, of course, accepted the charge and went on to reform conditions of filth, neglect, and want, improving the mortality of British wounded from 42.7 percent to 2.25 percent in a six-month period. She became known as the "Lady of the Lamp" for her practice of visiting the sickest of the wounded after her regular work was completed.

She had many difficulties to overcome, not the least of which was resistance to her leadership, because she was a civilian and female and because her authority circumvented that of the usual military hierarchy. She was effective in using all the sources of power available to her to make the revolutionary changes in military nursing practices.

Afterward, despite continuing ill health associated with her contraction of Crimean Fever, she worked to advance the cause of nursing, writing many books and articles and establishing the Nightingale Training School for Nurses.

Great Man Theories

Early studies of leadership focused on the traits demonstrated by acknowledged leaders in contrast to traits of those not acknowledged as leaders. This school of thought was called the trait, or Great Man, theory of leadership, and looked at the individual physical, psychological, or spiritual characteristics that differentiated born leaders from followers. Using this theory, one would explain Florence Nightingale's leadership as the result of inborn traits that predestined her to this role. Traits frequently thought to be associated with leadership included intelligence, physical prowess, dependability, sociability, and popularity (Stogdill, 1948).

One variant of the Great Man theory of leadership was the charismatic theory, which held that leaders are those who possess charisma or an attraction to which followers respond with fervor and commitment. Although it is evident that some people possess this rather undefinable and certainly unmeasurable trait, it was hard to find useful application for this theory, particularly because charisma is not always experienced by followers uniformly. Looking at Florence Nightingale through the eyes of charismatic theory, one would say that she inspired the nurses and others who worked with her by the strength of her vision and personality. The fact is, however, that Nightingale was not not seen as a charismatic leader by many influential people who assisted her work. They supported her not because she inspired them, but because she wielded social and political power.

The trait theory approach had a number of problems, because, as we have discussed, leaders in one situation may function as followers in another. In addition, leaders who were effective in some circumstances calling for sociability, popularity, and dependability were ineffective in others that required different characteristics. It became clear during the

1950s that trait theory alone was not enough to explain or predict leadership, and more important, did not supply useful information on how to develop leadership skills.

Another problem with focusing only on the characteristics of the leader is that it ignores the fact that leaders operate in groups. Behaviorist theories developed to describe leadership behavior in terms of both the qualities of the leader and the characteristics, abilities, and needs of the group.

During the 1970s there was a reappraisal of trait theory research that focused on the relationship of leader traits to leader effectiveness, rather than on the comparison of leaders to nonleaders. This proved to be a more productive approach and focused on the role of personality characteristics in leadership effectiveness. It acknowledges the contribution individual traits may play in the emergence of leaders in any given situation.

Situational Theories

As a reaction to the early trait theories another school of thought developed that initially focused on the other principal component of leadership, the situation in which the leader functions. Researchers focused on characteristics of the organization, or the situation, to explain leadership effectiveness. This approach examined such things as the hierarchical structure of the organization, the atmosphere of the organization, and the characteristics of the leadership role and the follower role (Hoy & Miskell, 1987). In this approach Nightingale would be seen to be effective not because of her personal characteristics or abilities, but because of the situation during the Crimean War. The situation demanded someone with knowledge of the social and political realities of the time, as well as the requisite knowledge of nursing practice. This approach helped to explain how effective leaders in one instance might be ineffective in others, but it tended to ignore the role of individual characteristics or the fact that individuals can vary their approaches to situations.

Contingency Theory

The contingency approach was developed by Fred Fiedler during the 1960s. He described three components of any situation that must be included in an examination of leader effectiveness: (1) the nature of the leader–member relationship, (2) the structure of the task to be performed, and (3) the position power wielded by the leader. Fiedler (1967) identifies eight situations based on these three criteria, ranging from very favorable to unfavorable. If the leader–member relationship is one in which followers have respect and confidence in the leader, if the task is structured and there are a number of possible solutions, and if the leader

An Adaptation of Fiedler's Classification of Situational Favorableness

LEADER/MEMBER RELATIONSHIP	TASK STRUCTURE	LEADER POSITION POWER	DEGREE OF FAVORABLENESS	MOST EFFECTIVE LEADER
Good	Structured	High	Very favorable	TASK ORIENTED
Good	Structured	Low		
Good	Unstructured	High		
Good	Unstructured	Low	Moderate	RELATIONSHIP ORIENTED
Poor	Structured	High	Moderate	
Poor	Structured	Low		
Poor	Unstructured	High		
Poor	Unstructured	Low	Unfavorable	TASK ORIENTED

Display 2.1
Source: Adapted from Wayne C. Hoy and Cecil G. Miskel (1987) Formulation of Fielder's Classification of Situational Favorableness in Educational Administration: Theory, Research and Practice, New York: Random House.

has power because of the support of the overall organization, then the situation is probably the most favorable.

On the other hand, in a situation where the leader does not have the confidence of the followers, where the task to be accomplished is difficult and has few solutions, and where the organization in which they function is disinterested or does not support the leader, the situation is highly unfavorable. Fiedler noticed that in favorable situations, leaders who are task oriented are the most effective. In moderately favorable situations, leaders who are relationship oriented are most effective. In unfavorable situations, it is the task–oriented leader who once again is most effective.

Contingency theory would hold that Nightingale was an effective leader because she was supported by followers who believed so strongly in her leadership that they were willing to endure many difficulties and privations. She was able to find solutions to the many problems of supplies, distribution, and finances; and she was successful in enlisting the support of influential organizations and individuals, such as the Secretary of War, Sidney Herbert. She also appeared to vary her leadership style with the situation, becoming more directive and task oriented when confronted with unfavorable circumstances and more relationship oriented during periods of relative favorability.

Path–Goal Theory

Path–goal theory, often considered a type of contingency theory, focuses on the behavior of the leader in increasing the acceptance, satisfaction, and motivation of followers. Developed by Robert J. House (1971), the theory describes four types of leadership behavior:

1. *Directive leadership.* A nurse using directive leadership focuses on rules and policies, making expectations clear to subordinates and giving specific directions for the accomplishment of tasks.
2. *Achievement-oriented leadership.* A nurse using this style of leadership behavior concentrates on identifying challenging goals. Subordinates are viewed as capable workers who are expected to achieve these goals. In contrast to the first type of leader, who focuses on rules and policies, this leader focuses on achievement and excellence.
3. *Supportive leadership.* A nurse exercising supportive leadership is concerned primarily with providing encouragement to subordinates and seeks to create an environment in which they can function optimally.
4. *Participative leadership.* In this style of leadership, a nurse works with subordinates in coming to a decision about their joint responsibilities and takes into account their views in arriving at a solution.

Path–goal theory not only emphasized the importance of leader behavior being acceptable to subordinates, but emphasized that followers are more apt to function in a goal-directed manner if satisfaction of their own needs is tied to goal achievement. The leader functions to provide both structure and a supportive environment for subordinates. Path–goal theory might explain Nightingale's effectiveness by focusing on both her ability to provide structure and direction for her nurses and to create an environment where they could fulfill their own desires to care effectively for the wounded soldiers.

Additional Approaches

Other writers who have contributed to the discussion of leadership and management have included Blake and Mouton (1985), who developed the managerial grid system of assessing management, and Hersey and Blanchard (1982), who looked at the importance of maturity in subordinates. Vroom and Yetton (1973) developed models for making management decisions. They identified five methods of decision making, ranging from unilateral, with no participation by subordinates, to shared, in which the group itself makes the decision based upon information from the leader. They presented strategies to enhance both the quality of decisions and the acceptance of decisions.

One very popular application of management theory is termed *management by objectives,* or MBO. This management method focuses on the importance of establishing mutually supported goals. As Douglass and Bevis (1979) describe it, MBO philosophy recognizes that each person within an organization has internal as well as external, or organizational, controls over behavior. The more that individual needs and goals can be meshed with those of the organization, the more effective management will be.

The procedure for implementing MBO involves the establishment of goals, planning for implementation, actual implementation of the agreed-upon process, and evaluation of the results. The establishing of goals requires careful assessment of needs and resources of both individuals and the institution. Generally, this is done on an annual basis, and adequate time must be provided for this review. Using this information, goals and objectives are then identified, based upon the ability of the goal to contribute to the organization as a whole, the feasibility of accomplishing it, and the priority of need. Both long-term and short-term goals are established.

Planning for implementation involves establishing a time-line, identifying individual responsibilities, resources, settings, and methods. Only after this is done and agreed upon is implementation begun. Equally important is the assessment following implementation, which identifies whether goals have been achieved. If they have not been achieved, reasons for failure are identified, other courses of action and resources examined, and another approach or abandonment of the goal is decided upon.

The strength of the MBO approach is its ability to motivate all individuals involved. Managers and subordinates who jointly identify goals, work toward their accomplishment, and evaluate the results have a shared commitment that lends strength to the enterprise.

In Conclusion

Each theory of leadership makes a contribution to our understanding of this complex role. Clearly, a variety of variables contribute to effective leadership, including personal characteristics and situational characteristics. Effective leaders are those who acknowledge the importance of both task-oriented and relationship-oriented actions and seek to provide structure and support for subordinates.

APPROACHES TO ORGANIZATIONAL MANAGEMENT

There are three approaches to the examination of organizational management: classical organizational thought, the human relations approach, and the behavioral science approach. *Classical organizational thought* was an outgrowth of the work of Frederick Taylor during the early 1900s. Taylor saw his workers as cogs in a machine and concentrated on time management studies that allowed them to work faster and more efficiently. This approach maximized the importance of physiological factors and virtually ignored psychological and sociological considerations.

The *human relations approach* developed during the 1930s as the result of work by Mary Parker Follett, who examined the importance of relationships in organizations. The best-known studies based upon this approach were conducted at the Hawthorne electric plant by Mayo and Roethlisberger. During these studies the importance of interpersonal relations between supervisors and subordinates was demonstrated repeatedly and the role of social conditions in organizational effectiveness was identified. Workers could no longer simply be considered as cogs in a machine; their attitudes, their concerns, and their relationships were as important to effective operation as their physical abilities.

The *behavioral science approach* developed during the 1950s. The researchers most closely identified with it are Chester Barnard and Herbert Simon. This approach went another step further in analyzing organizational effectiveness by examining the contribution of social relations and formal structure in interaction. Barnard looked at both the formal and informal structures that exist in any organization and identified additional components such as the cooperative system that must be a part of any organizational assessment.

Herbert Simon described the organization as an exchange system in which employees produced work for specific inducements as long as they perceived the inducements as more substantial than the effort required. Simon felt that there were no ideal solutions to management problems but that some could be seen as more satisfactory than others. This principle of "satisficing," or arriving at mutually satisfying solutions, meant that effective decisions could be reached in which the participants saw the results as individually beneficial.

TYPES OF MANAGEMENT

Individual characteristics constitute one important variable that determines the type of manager a nurse might be. Another, of course, is the type of institutional organization in which the nurse functions. In the preceding chapter you became acquainted with various types of organizations. The degree to which authority is centralized or dispersed and the way in which communication and consultation occur have great influence on the type of manager a nurse will be. In addition, the nurse manager can choose to focus on the tasks to be done, on the motivation and satisfaction of the subordinates, or on a combination of approaches. Within the constraints of leadership style and organizational structure, three basic management types can be described: authoritarian, democratic, and laissez-faire.

Authoritarian Management Style

The authoritarian, or autocratic, manager tends to make most decisions in isolation. Although subordinates may volunteer suggestions, authoritarian managers do not necessarily take them into consideration, because they feel that they are in a better position to understand the whole situation. Authoritarian managers are characteristically found in bureaucratic organizations that reinforce the centrality of authority and reliance upon formal rules. Authoritarian managers issue orders and expect to be obeyed. Their authority generally derives from position power that is tied to their official hierarchical title.

Disadvantages of this type of management style are clear. If subordinates feel they are not listened to or supported, they are less likely to have a personal stake in the achievement of management goals. Although they may be coerced into following the orders of the manager, they may indirectly subvert these goals. Advantages of this style of management include the fact that decisions can be made expeditiously without the lengthy time required for consultation and arriving at a collaboratively agreed-upon course of action.

Authoritarian management is appropriate when there is a need for immediate action and the manager is the individual with the best understanding of the situation. An example of this type of management might occur in an emergency room setting.

> Nurse Brown is the emergency room nurse on Thursday evening, working with a receptionist, an EMT, and the ER physician, Dr. Black. In the waiting room at 9:00 P.M. is a mother with a young child complaining of earache, a teenager who has cut his hand hitting a window, and, just arriving, an older gentleman who is in obvious distress. His face is pale and his skin is clammy, but he dismisses his discomfort as indigestion. The EMT begins to take the bleeding teenager back to a treatment room. The mother of the young child protests that she was here first. The receptionist announces that it is time for her supper break and prepares to leave for the cafeteria.
>
> Nurse Brown, because of his position as leader of the group and because of his greater knowledge of the possible ramifications of each patient's presenting symptomatology, takes charge of the situation in an authoritarian style. He orders the EMT to take the older gentleman into the cardiac assessment room and the receptionist to call Dr. Black first and then to call the cardiopulmonary technician and the laboratory technician. He prepares to start an IV, to draw blood samples, and to attach EKG leads on the older gentleman.

This situation is one in which an authoritarian leader functions best.

The leader is in the best position to make judgments and decisions. There is not time to explain to subordinates why things must be accomplished, and there is not time to allow for discussion of alternative approaches. Because of his authority, Nurse Brown's orders will be followed, and a possible myocardial infarction will be dealt with expeditiously.

After the patient is admitted to the intensive care unit for further observation, Nurse Brown takes time to thank his staff for their prompt response and does some teaching regarding early signs of myocardial infarction. He assists his staff in making explanations to the rest of the patients and in seeing that they are appropriately cared for.

Authoritarian managers will continue to have the full support of their subordinates only if they are able to involve them in the overall goals and processes. Given the nature of the emergency room, this may have to be done at times other than when decisions are actually being made. By recognizing the contribution of subordinates and by assisting them to increase their own skills and knowledge, managers help to ensure that their authority is maintained and that their orders will be effectively followed in the future.

Democratic Management Style

The democratic manager, in contrast to the authoritarian manager, focuses on involving subordinates in decision making. In contrast to relying upon hierarchical authority, the democratic managers see themselves as coworkers, rather than as superiors, and stress the importance of communication and consensus. Although the manager may hold a position of higher authority, this authority is not exercised in a coercive manner, and the manager leads by providing information, suggesting direction, and being supportive of coworkers. Generally, the democratic manager functions best in an organization where power is less centralized and where there is less reliance on formal rules and policies.

Disadvantages of this style of management are that decision making can become a lengthy process. In addition, if coworkers are not confident about their own abilities to participate in planning and decision making, they may feel that the manager is not doing his or her job and is foisting difficult decisions off onto others who are not being paid to manage. Further, if decisions of the group cannot be implemented, coworkers may feel that the time and effort invested have been wasted.

Advantages of the democratic style are that coworkers who are consulted and who have input into decisions are more motivated to support such decisions. Involving subordinates in the data gathering, analysis, planning, implementation, and evaluation of tasks ensures the widest possible scope and may provide information to which the manager alone would not have had access.

Democratic management is appropriate when the task or decision at hand is not one that requires urgent action, when subordinates can be expected to make meaningful contributions, and when their input can be taken into account. An example of democratic management might occur on a medical surgical floor.

Nurse Smith is working with a newly graduated nurse, an LPN, and a nursing assistant. Together they have responsibility for medical patients in one wing of Hammerton Hospital. Nurse Smith has confidence in her subordinates, having worked with them previously. She knows that they are keen observers and often bring her important information about their patients. She knows also that they function within their assigned roles and are careful not to exceed their authority.

As they report for duty, Nurse Smith and her subordinates receive report on their group of patients. Following report, they meet to formulate a plan to deliver care. Nurse Smith requests their input, particularly on patients they might have cared for previously. LPN Jones indicates that one patient has to be watched particularly closely because of a tendency to climb over the bed rails. Nursing Assistant White suggests that another patient might be a particularly interesting assignment for the new graduate nurse, because the patient has a condition that is rarely seen at this hospital. The four coworkers design a plan for jointly caring for the assigned patients, with the team manager, Nurse Smith, providing information, encouragement, and direction as it is needed.

Laissez-Faire Management Style

Also called *permissive management,* laissez-faire management provides the least structure and control. It requires coworkers to develop their own goals, make their own decisions, and take responsibility for their own management. Managers concentrate on providing maximum support and freedom for coworkers.

Disadvantages of this style in most health care settings are numerous. Generally, it is not possible to let each coworker arrive at an individual approach to decisions about patients. Because of the multidisciplinary nature of patient care, there generally must be more centralized decision making and agreement in following generally accepted policies and procedures.

Advantages of this style of management include providing maximum freedom for individuals and, presumably, a resulting increased motivation of subordinates to perform at high levels because of this independence. An example of laissez-faire management might occur in an inpatient psychiatric unit.

Nurse Stevens is one of four registered nurses who provides care to established patients on an inpatient psychiatric unit. The supervising nurse, recognizing the competence and responsibility of the four RNs, allows them individually to structure and deliver care for the patients for whom they are responsible as long as general schedules for meals, group meetings, and medication administration are adhered to. Each nurse develops an individual plan of care in conjunction with the individual patient. The progress of each patient is shared with other members of the staff by the registered nurse at regularly scheduled case conference meetings at which the psychiatrist, the social services worker, and other professionals also present information.

In circumstances where a laissez-faire approach to management is inappropriately attempted, a leadership vacuum may occur. In these instances it is not uncommon for an informal leader to arise who will give direction to the group. Coworkers recognize an implicit authority or degree of expertise in the informal leader. This may temporarily allow the group to continue to function while the informal leader provides the necessary direction and assistance.

Multicratic Leadership

Each of the three management styles may be used effectively, depending upon the situation involved. One of the skills of leadership is identifying which style of management a particular situation requires. This so-called *multicratic approach* combines the best of all approaches, mediated by the requirements of the situation at hand. For the new graduate, learning which is the best approach requires study and practice, as is the case with other nursing skills. The multicratic leader provides a maximum of structure when the situation requires it, a maximum of group participation when this is needed, and support and encouragement for subordinates in all instances.

Nonproductive Management Styles

Although any of the three management styles mentioned above can be used inappropriately in certain circumstances, some styles of management are nearly always harmful. These include the manager as Sacrificial Lamb, the manager as High Priestess/Priest, and the manager as Mother.

Manager as Sacrificial Lamb

In the first nonproductive style, the manager sees himself or herself as ennobled because of continual self-sacrifice. This manager is apt to stay overtime to finish up unit work, take schedules home to work on over the weekend, or arrive early to see that the inventory has been done properly. These managers generally feel that subordinates cannot be entirely trusted to do things acceptably, and that their own status is enhanced by their willingness to put in extra time and effort. This manager can be a productive one as long as everyone supports the necessary fiction and

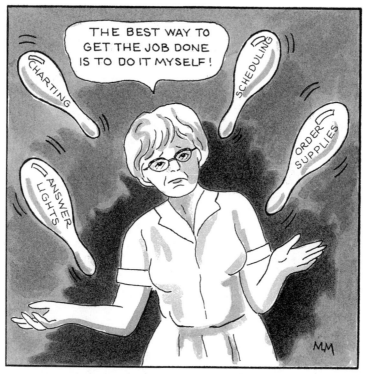

The manager as Sacrificial Lamb generally feels that her status is enhanced by her willingness to put in extra time.

colleagues reward the manager with appreciation or recognition. If colleagues attempt to rectify the situation by assuming more individual responsibility, the manager frequently responds in a hostile manner.

Suggestions for new graduates who find themselves working with a manager masquerading as Sacrificial Lamb include making certain that assistance from the manager is appropriately acknowledged and working to enlist the interest and support of the manager in the development of the new graduate. If these managers can be encouraged to assist in the process of orientation and teaching, they are often very dedicated and hardworking. In the long run, developing a relationship in which the subordinate can assume proper responsibility without the need for a self-sacrificing superior is important.

Manager as High Priestess/Priest

High priestess/priest managers see themselves as ministering to some higher authority, either the organization itself or another entity such as the medical staff. A manager who sees the corporation as the supreme entity will interpret management decisions in light of the corporate good.

A manager who sees the physician as paramount and infallible will usually defer to the medical leadership. In this style of management, communication occurs from the top down, with the High Priest or Priestess interpreting the dictates from corporate administration or medical staff. Because their status depends on being able to serve in this ministering function, these managers are often reluctant to share information, because this might dilute their authority. Information on physician preferences or corporate policies is not shared openly, but pronouncements based upon them serve as the basis for ongoing management.

Suggestions for new graduates in working with this type of manager include recognizing that you will probably learn more about individual physician preferences from the doctor in question and more about institutional policies from other experienced nursing staff. You should avoid threatening the manager, because such managers are not noted for welcoming the opportunity to share the limelight with others. Legitimately recognizing their knowledge and expertise may help to make the new graduate's relationship with this manager more congenial.

Manager as Mother

Like the previous two nonproductive managers, the manager as Mother sees coworkers and subordinates as basically unable to function independently. This manager, however, focuses efforts on nurturing and usually overprotecting subordinates, thwarting their development as autonomous professionals. Communications to subordinates from others are indirect and mediated through the Mother, who often alters them to make messages more dilute and less "threatening." The manager as Mother spends much time helping to perform subordinates' tasks rather than teaching self-reliance and organizational skills necessary for independent functioning.

This manager is often well liked by staff, who see the individual as very supportive and "willing to pitch in and help." It's only when this excessive support and protection are missing that it becomes evident that subordinates have not been assisted to grow into fully functioning coworkers and effective followers.

Often this type of manager is an easy one for new graduates to work with. A good initial relationship can be established if acknowledgment is given for the assistance and expertise of the manager. As the graduate gains independence and seeks more responsibility, care must be taken to avoid open rejection of mothering by the manager. Often, if couched in terms of assisting the new graduate to develop new organizational skills, the increasing independence desired can be obtained without alienating the manager. A frank discussion of goals and needs is frequently helpful. If you as a new graduate can enlist the support of the manager in develop-

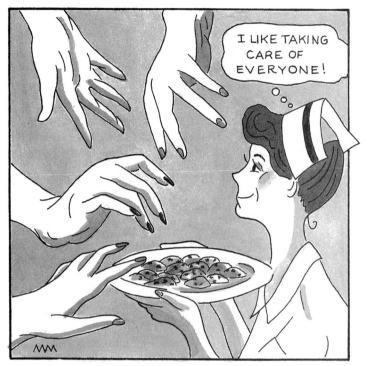

The manager as Mother focuses efforts on nurturing and usually overprotects subordinates.

ing your own capacities and skills, this frequently leads to a change in the relationship in which a healthier manager–subordinate interaction can occur.

THE RECIPROCAL ROLE: BEING A GOOD FOLLOWER

Billye Brown (1980) has pointed out that there are two parties to any leadership situation: the leader and follower. Frequently, followers are incorrectly viewed as merely passive recipients of management strategies who carry out directives or who fail to do so. In reality, each role has responsibilities and expectations, and each individual is an active agent within the relationship. As Brown points out, the effective follower is able to perceive a relationship between the institutional goals and personal goals and views the leader as working toward the accomplishment of both. She further suggests that the characteristics associated with leadership are also necessary in followership, used in different degrees in different settings. She also points out that leader and follower roles are frequently interchanged.

The importance of recognizing this interchanging of roles in today's health care settings is great. Registered nurses who are expected to manage the care of patients at the bedside and to lead subordinates who support them in this process are also expected to be competent followers of nurse specialists, supervisors, and administrators.

As a new graduate there are several ways to ensure that you assume an effective follower role:

1. *Invest yourself.* When you made a decision regarding employment, you did so because you saw the opportunity to accomplish your own goals and objectives. Perhaps the organization specializes in caring for a particular type of patient with whom you are interested in working. Perhaps the institution has the reputation of delivering excellent nursing care. Whatever the motivation that prompted you to accept your new position, you must begin to see how your own goals fit into the goals of the larger organization, whether this is viewed as the nursing service or the organization as a whole. To the degree that they are congruent, you will feel more of an investment in your role as follower. If you discover that there is a fundamental conflict between organizational goals and your personal goals, it may be necessary for you to reevaluate your decision to work there, because this may substantially compromise your ability to be an effective follower or leader. (See Chapter 3 for a further discussion of goal setting.)

2. *Clearly identify your responsibilities as a follower.* What is expected of you, to whom do you report, how is your performance evaluated? Only by knowing specifically what your role is will you be able to fulfill it. As a new graduate you will be using your orientation time to learn your new role. Usual resources will include your job description, the procedure manual for the unit on which you will be working, and policies dealing with institutional functioning, including evaluation and training of workers. During the orientation process make certain you identify the resource person to whom you can go for continued clarification and assistance during the period following the orientation.

3. *Clearly identify your expectations of the leader.* Ensure that you understand this individual's role and relationship to you. Just as you must be cognizant of your own responsibilities, you need to understand what to expect realistically from your leader in relation to you and other members of the group. If you hold unrealistic expectations of the leader, this may compromise your ability to perform your own role effectively and may make it difficult to establish an appropriate relationship with this leader.

4. *Support your leader and your group.* Once you are committed to jointly held goals and have a clear understanding of your role as follower and the manager's role as leader, work toward the effective functioning of your group. This may sound as if it is self-evident, but unfortunately it is not uncommon for nurses to feel that their only obligation is to patients directly in their charge. Learning to work productively with others to achieve patient care goals is a much more effective way of ensuring that goals for all patients are met.

5. *Challenge your leader and your group.* One of the most important services followers can provide is to stimulate discussion, to provide a fresh look at problems, and to propose other potential solutions. Obviously, this is most effective when done in a constructive manner and with the support of the leader and group. Effective followers are not merely compliant subordinates, but rather coworkers who see a personal responsibility in maintaining the best possible work environment.

6. *Follow channels of communication and responsibility.* As a new graduate you should be oriented to the organizational structure, with channels of authority and routes of communication. Although you may be tempted to take questions or problems to the most sympathetic coworker or leader, it is important to follow established channels. This ensures that the leader involved is aware of the concern, and it also serves to hold the leader responsible for a constructive response. Only when this is not forthcoming should an approach be made to someone further up the chain of authority, and generally it is best to inform the immediate leader of your intent to contact this person. Only if leaders are held accountable can authority be effectively managed; followers as well as managers have responsibility for ensuring that this is the case.

Nonproductive Followers

Just as leaders can assume nonproductive management styles, followers can adopt unhelpful ways of interacting with managers. You may see some examples of nonproductive followership.

Appliance Nurses

The so-called *appliance nurses* are those who declare themselves "only in it for the money," who are interested solely in the necessities or conveniences wages can buy.

Although all of us must understand the importance of adequate payment for nurses, there is much more to a professional commitment than working for a wage. Followers who see their responsibility only in terms of hours and paychecks are less likely to be fully functioning members with a view of the larger picture. Nurses at all levels must be involved in maintaining current practice, in participating in professional organizations and self-governance, and in serving as advocates for those needing nursing services. Nurses who see their responsibilities ending with the completion of the shift are minimizing the contribution they can make as effective followers or leaders.

Doomsayers

The incurable pessimist has a vested interest in portraying the situation as one without solution; if there is no solution to any given problem, then individuals cannot be held accountable for failures. Doomsayers bemoan the lack of supplies, the shortness of staff, the insensitivity of management, or other difficulties without attempting to suggest solutions or to work for change. These followers are very difficult to work with because each attempt by the leader or group to improve the situation merely meets with a different explanation for why the suggested innovation will be insufficient.

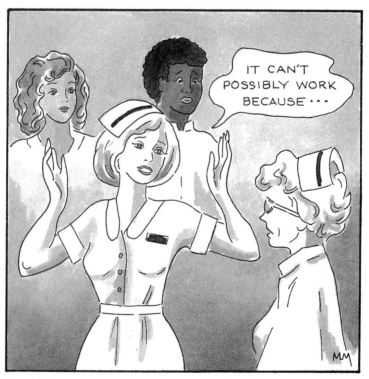

The incurable pessimist has a vested interest in portraying the situation as one without solutions.

This is not to suggest that followers should blindly accept a situation to avoid negativity, but it does point out that as a member of a profession, each nurse is responsible for contributing to finding solutions to problems. Working with Doomsayers requires reeducation to show these individuals that their input is valued and can result in productive change.

Subversives

Subversives are followers who take pessimism one step further, consciously or unconsciously undermining the leader or group. Frequently, these followers feel disappointed with their own situation and seek to exert some measure of control by exercising their power to subvert the goals of the leader and group. Occasionally, they have an antipathy to authority figures whom they suspect of some organizational bias that must be guarded against. An example of a Subversive in action might be seen in a situation where new charting forms are being introduced. Although some nurses are enthusiastic about the change and others are concerned about making the change, the Subversive engineers a plot to defeat the new forms without a trial by encouraging others to fill them out improperly or not to fill them out at all, substituting the original forms instead.

Working with subversive followers is difficult, because any administrator may be viewed by definition as unreliable, or sold out to organizational interests (Sullivan & Decker, 1988). Persistent demonstration of concern for subordinates may help to mitigate this suspicion and reduce the amount of subversion. Frank discussion of the follower's nonproductive action or inaction is also important.

Accommodators

Just as followers who always oppose the leader are difficult with whom to work, so are followers who always accommodate to that individual. Followers have responsibility for providing feedback to leaders in a consistent and positive manner. If they neglect this responsibility and simply accommodate to avoid having to confront or provide negative feedback, the leader is less able to function effectively. Learning to be an assertive follower is just as important as learning not to be obstructionist. An example of an accommodator is the staff person who fails to voice concerns about the new leader's plans to take over all scheduling responsibilities for the unit. The staff person knows that this task is viewed by her coworkers as an important shared responsibility. Rather than voice these concerns, the accommodator prefers simply to "go along," not making waves, with the result that the new leader makes a decision without information that could be helpful.

DEVELOPING YOUR OWN MANAGEMENT STYLE

Each person will develop an individual management style. The following will help you explore ways to make your management style effective.

Self-assessment

You already have developed a style of working with both leaders and followers. Begin to analyze the ways in which you interact with others, including fellow students, instructors, nursing staff, and patients. Do you find that you are more comfortable in situations where you are told precisely what is expected? In this case, as a follower you may feel more comfortable in a bureaucratic organizational structure in which the leader utilizes an authoritarian management style. When you relate to other students in groups, do you feel more comfortable when members all have a voice in the operation of the group? Do you feel that group members ought to be unfettered by constraints? If so, you may feel more comfortable with democratic or permissive management styles. Obviously, your preferences will depend to some extent on the situation in question, but developing an awareness of your comfort level with the various styles of management will provide important background data for you.

Environmental Assessment

Just as important as a knowledge of self is a knowledge of the work environment. Assess the nature of the unit and the hospital in which you will be working. Based upon what you know of the relative advantages and disadvantages of different management styles in different work environments, begin to identify those that might be most productive in this setting.

Identification of Role Models

You have most likely observed nurses functioning as leaders and followers whom you feel are particularly effective. Begin to look more closely at their operating styles. How do they interact with subordinates and superiors? How do they involve coworkers in activities with joint responsibilities? What communication strategies do they utilize? What bases of power do they access? Frequently, these effective managers are quite willing to talk about their approach to followers and can provide very helpful suggestions to new nurses. Practice using the worksheet in the display to examine the management style of nurses you might wish to emulate. You can also use the worksheet to help you analyze your own management skills and style as these develop. An effective management

Management Skills Worksheet

Identify a nurse whose management style you would like to emulate. Observe the ways this person interacts with subordinates, coworkers, and superiors. Attempt to identify when your role model uses an authoritarian approach, democratic, or laissez-faire approach in the following situations. Note skills and techniques you might like to consider in developing your own management style.

Description of Situation

Management Skill	Management Style or Technique	Effectiveness
Setting goals		
Using power		
Managing resources		
Decision making		
Managing time		
Developing motivation		
Teaching staff		
Using feedback		
Managing conflict		
Advocating effectively		
Using research		

Notes

style makes use of the skills and techniques discussed in subsequent chapters and includes setting goals and objectives, understanding and using power, managing resources, making decisions, managing time, developing motivation, teaching staff, using feedback, managing conflict, and serving as an effective advocate.

Trying Out Management Styles

All the observation, data gathering, and assessment of management styles is ineffective if it is not put into action. After you have assessed yourself, assessed your environment, and identified a management style you feel you would like to emulate, practice utilizing it in your work responsibility. If this means a change from your current operating style, it is usually helpful to inform subordinates or coworkers that you are trying something different and to enlist their assistance. If this means a move to a more democratic structure, it may be important to make clear to subordinates exactly what their responsibilities will be under the new system. If, for example, you as the registered nurse were accustomed to assigning subordinates responsibilities without input from them and wished to begin incorporating their information, it would be important to let them know that you will expect such input, that it will be used in making decisions about assignments, and that you value their participation. As a new nurse, you may find the management skills worksheet helpful in beginning to explore your own approach to management. You may use it to evaluate the management skills of nurses you observe and to keep track of management strategies you yourself try out.

Evaluating Effectiveness

Just as with any other nursing intervention, evaluation of the effectiveness of your management style is important, particularly during the formative period or periods of change. Identify specifically the characteristics of your management style on which you want feedback. Do you want to know if communications are effective? if decision making is expeditious? if subordinates feel consulted and valued? Requesting specific information on these aspects of your management style will assist you to make ongoing adjustments and to develop a style of management that is effective for you and the group.

SUMMARY

Fawcett and Carino (1989), in their discussion of hallmarks of success in nursing practice, identify as one of the emerging hallmarks changes in nursing care delivery systems. They point to the important development of case management approaches and other approaches growing out of primary nursing structures as evidence of substantive progress in nursing practice. In both these approaches, management, whether practiced by the supervising nurse or the nurse at the bedside, is crucial. Further, the use of conceptual models to guide nursing practice—another important hallmark of nursing success—presupposes a coordinating, directing role that can only be expected to increase as nursing assumes its full responsibility in the delivery of patient care.

In this chapter we have looked at management as a component of the leadership role. Examples of theories about leadership, including trait theory, behaviorist theory, and situational theory have been discussed. We have looked at contingency theory and at path goal theory as one recent extension of contingency theory. Each makes a contribution to our understanding of how effective leadership involves characteristics of leaders, followers, and the situation in which they function. We have seen how effective leaders vary their style with the demands of the situation, providing both structure and support to subordinates.

We have examined three main management styles, along with their advantages and disadvantages. We have looked at examples of situations in which authoritarian management, democratic management, and laissez-faire management each might be productively used. Because nurses function as both leaders and followers, we have also examined the role of follower and the characteristics of effective and ineffective followership.

Finally, we have made suggestions on beginning to develop your own effective management style, beginning with an assessment of your own leadership and followership characteristics. An assessment of the work environment, the identification of good role models, the experimentation with different styles, and the evaluation of their effectiveness are all part of the ongoing process of developing a good management style.

Perhaps the most crucial point in this chapter is that all registered nurses, regardless of position, must be prepared to function as managers. Although this aspect of the leadership role may not come as comfortably as learning psychomotor skill competencies in a particular clinical setting, the fact that nurses are responsible for coordinating and managing care of patients, for delegating tasks to subordinates, and for supervising that activity means that nurses must be prepared to function as managers. You as a new nurse must exercise the same diligence and commitment in learning these skills as you expect to do in other professional areas.

Study Questions Activities

1. What aspects of leadership are emphasized by the Great Man theory of leadership?
2. In contrast to trait theory, how does situational theory explain the emergence of leaders?

3. What are the three components used in contingency theory to explain the favorableness or nonfavorableness of any leadership situation?

4. How do the four types of leaders described by House differ?

5. In what situations is authoritarian management appropriate? democratic management? laissez-faire management?

6. What are examples of nonproductive management styles?

7. What are examples of nonproductive follower styles? productive styles?

8. How would you go about finding out which management style might be most effective for you?

9. Why is it important for staff nurses to learn about leadership and management?

REFERENCES

Blake, R.R., & Mouton, J.S. (1985). *The managerial grid III.* Houston: Gulf.

Brown, B. (1980). Follow the leader. *Nursing Outlook, 28*(6), 357–359.

Donahue, M.P. (1985). *Nursing: the finest art.* St. Louis: C.V. Mosby.

Douglass, L.M., & Bevis, E.M. (1979). *Nursing management and leadership in action.* St. Louis: C.V. Mosby.

Fawcett, J., & Carino, C. (1989). Hallmarks of success in nursing practice. *Advances in Nursing Science, 11*(4), 1–8.

Fiedler, F.E. (1967). *A theory of leadership effectiveness.* New York: McGraw-Hill.

Hersey, P., & Blanchard, K.H. (1982). *Management of organizational behavior: Utilizing human resources,* 4th ed. Englewood Cliffs, N.J.: Prentice-Hall.

House, R.J. (1971). A path-goal theory of leadership effectiveness. *Administrative Science Quarterly, 16,* 321–338.

Hoy, W.K., and Miskel, C.G. (1987). *Educational administration: Theory, research and practice.* New York: Random House.

Kaler, S.R., Levy, D.A., & Schall, M. (1989). Stereotypes of professional roles. *Image, 21*(2), 85–89.

O'Grady, T.M. (1989). Shared governance: Reality or sham? *American Journal of Nursing, 89*(3), 350–351.

Stogdill, R.M. (1948). Personal factors associated with leadership: A survey of the literature. *Journal of Psychology, 25,* 35–71.

Stogdill, R.M. (1950). Leadership, membership, and organization. *Psychological Bulletin, 47,* 4.

Storfjell, J.L. (1989). How valuable are nurses' skills? A case for fair pricing in home health care. *Nursing & Health Care, 10*(6), 311–313.

Sullivan, E.J., & Decker, P.J. (1988). *Effective management in nursing.* Reading, Mass.: Addison-Wesley.

Vroom, V.H., & Yetton, P.W. (1973). *Leadership and decision making.* Pittsburgh: University of Pittsburgh Press.

Woodham-Smith, C. (1951). *Florence Nightingale.* New York: McGraw-Hill.

SUGGESTIONS FOR FURTHER READING

Chenevert, M. (1985). *Pro-nurse handbook*. St Louis: C.V. Mosby.

Dossett, D.L., Jenkins, R.L., Decker, P.J., & Sullivan, E.J. (1988). Leadership skills. In E.J. Sullivan & P.J. Decker, Eds. *Effective management in nursing*. Reading, Mass.: Addison-Wesley.

French, W.L., Kast, F.E., & Rosenzweig, J.E. (1985). *Understanding human behavior in organizations*. New York: Harper & Row.

Gambacorta, S. (1983). Head nurses face reality shock too! *Nursing Management, 14*(7), 46.

Hein, E.C., & Nicholson, M.J. (1986). *Contemporary leadership behavior: Selected readings*. Boston: Little, Brown & Co.

Jenkins, R.L., & Henderson, R.L. (1984). Motivating the staff: What nurses expect from their supervisors. *Nursing Management, 15*(2), 13.

Johnston, P.F. (1983). Improving the nurse-physician relationship. *Journal of Nursing Administration, 13*(3), 19.

La Monica, E. (1983). *Nursing leadership and management: An experimental approach*. Monterey, Calif.: Wadsworth Health Sciences Division.

Levenstein, A. (1985). Caught in the middle. *Nursing Management, 16*(7), 46.

Luthans, F. (1985). *Organizational behavior*. New York: McGraw-Hill.

McGee, R.F. (1984). Leadership styles: A survey. *Nursing Success Today, 1*, 26.

Moloney, M.M. (1970). *Leadership in nursing: Theory, strategies, action*. St. Louis: C.V. Mosby.

Naisbit, J. (1982). *Megatrends*. New York: Warner Books.

Robey, D. (1986). *Designing organizations*. Homewood, Ill.: Irwin.

Thompson, A.M., & Wood, M.D. (1980). *Management strategies for women*. New York: Simon & Schuster.

Veninga, R.L. (1987). When bad things happen to good nursing departments: How to stay hopeful in tough times. *Journal of Nursing Administration, 17*(2), 35–40.

Establishing and Evaluating Goals

Objectives

After completing this chapter, you should be able to

1. *Distinguish between goals and objectives.*
2. *Identify the purpose of goals and objectives in a nursing arena.*
3. *Write professional goals and objectives for a nursing unit, shift of duty, or specific group of clients.*
4. *Discuss the behaviors that may characterize goal displacement.*
5. *Describe the importance of congruence between your professional philosophy and that of a current or potential employer.*
6. *Identify the use of goals and objectives in the evaluation process.*
7. *Relate goals and objectives of a nursing team or unit to the hospital quality assurance program.*

Many nurses react with dismay to the suggestion that they learn about or actually write goals and objectives. An often heard comment is, "That is for educators, not me. After all, I am a clinical manager." However, the truth is that everyone needs goals and objectives as a method of managing everyday life. Personal goals may not be clearly spelled out or well stated, but they may serve the individual. However, without clear goals in a care setting it will be difficult for everyone to be focused in the same direction and to work together effectively.

A major concept of clinical management is that of planning. According to Douglass (1988), determining goals and objectives is the initial step in the planning process. The art of establishing goals that positively influence the quality of care given to a professional's clients needs to be taught, learned, and practiced.

DEFINING GOALS AND OBJECTIVES

Goals are the broad statements of overall intent of an organization or individual. They are usually stated in general terms. *Objectives* are the

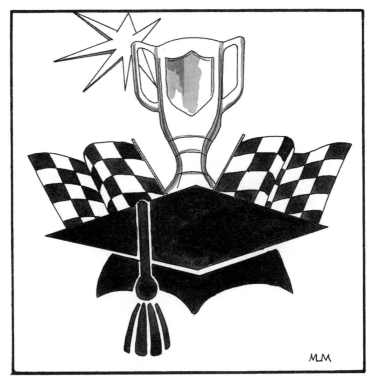

Goals stated in specific and measurable terms help us realize when the intent is achieved.

specific accomplishments that indicate the goal has been met. It is easy to conceptualize the goal as the umbrella and the objectives as the spines of the umbrella that allow it to function.

WRITING GOALS AND OBJECTIVES

The purpose of writing goals is to identify where you are going and to enable you to evaluate when you have arrived there. It is generally not effective to try to operate with goals and objectives that are not clearly written and openly shared.

Basically, a meaningfully stated goal is one that succeeds in communicating the intent of those generating the goal. It should be stated in such a way that it will be understood clearly by others. As in all communication, there is a risk of error in understanding. Many words used in goal writing are open to a variety of interpretations if definitions are not carefully spelled out. Other words are open to fewer interpretations. Table 3–1 points out examples of both types of terms. These lists are included to give you an example or point of reference for writing goals and objectives and are not meant to be an exclusive prescription.

The chief rule for writing goals is quite simple: Write them so they can be understood. That is it! Write your goals so their meaning is clear and so that they do not contain fuzzy words or thoughts. Some examples of nonfuzzy goals and objectives as they might relate to a student and to a client follow.

STUDENT

Goal: Complete psychology 101 with an "A" grade.
Objectives

1. Attend 95 percent of lectures.
2. Read 100 percent of chapters.
3. Achieve 92 percent or above on all tests.

CLIENT

Goal: Perform insulin self-injection using proper technique.
Objectives

1. Listen to 100 percent of instructions given by nurse.
2. Watch 100 percent of demonstrations given by nurse.
3. Perform return demonstrations supervised by the nurse until able to perform self-injection using proper technique.

TABLE 3–1. TERMS USED IN STATING GOALS

Words Open to Many Interpretations

To know
To understand
To really understand
To appreciate
To fully appreciate
To grasp the significance of
To enjoy
To believe
To have faith in

Words Open to Fewer Interpretations

To write
To demonstrate
To identify
To differentiate
To solve
To construct
To list
To compare
To contrast

(Mager, R.F. [1962]. *Preparing instructional objectives.* Belmont, Calif., Fearon Publishers)

The ability to make decisions develops when the nurse has clearly defined priorities that are based upon well-written and achievable goals (Sullivan & Decker, 1983). The more measurable the goal, the more likely it is that action will be taken toward its accomplishment and the less likely that it will be distorted.

The more you work with this process, the more easily you will recall it when you are required to determine priorities in the clinical area. On the most hectic day of the week, when you must make decisions quickly and effectively, the real value of goals and objectives will be clear to you.

GOALS AND OBJECTIVES IN NURSING PRACTICE

As a nurse in a health care institution, you need to be aware of the existence of several levels of goals: the institutional level, the nursing department level, and the nursing unit level. These goal levels all need to relate to the health needs of the community, because these are the focus of health care.

Institutional Goals

Based on the community's health needs, the institution forms goals and objectives. To take a current health care problem as an example, some communities are large enough that there is an expressed need for bone marrow transplant services. Based on this need, the hospital Board of Trustees might appoint a task force to study the question and gather the information necessary for making a decision. If the information gathered reveals that this need is great enough to support a program, the Board might set an institutional goal to have a fully staffed, inpatient bone marrow transplant program within 2 years. The board would then determine specific objectives and communicate the goals and objectives to each level of the institution's hierarchy. This communication is essential for an effective response by management.

An institution that focuses thinking on goals for the future and activities that will move the organization toward these goals is referred to as a *proactive* institution. The administrators of such institutions spend a great deal of time, money, and energy on identifying possible future events and

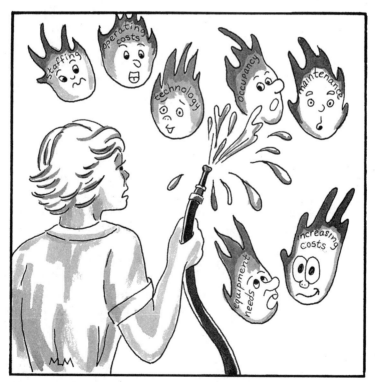

Institutions that do not have futuristic goals spend their time reacting to events and "putting out fires."

on preparing the institution to deal with them. An example of a proactive facility is one that plans for a nursing shortage by establishing scholarship funds for employees who desire to become nurses or that plans for the impact of AIDS by planning strategies to incorporate care of persons with that disease. Institutions that do not have specific or future-oriented goals are *reactive* institutions. They spend their time reacting to events, that is, "putting out fires" rather than "preventing them." A reactive facility would wait until such emergencies occurred and then would handle them as a crisis rather than as an anticipated event.

Nursing Department Goals

The goals of the institution definitely impact on those of nursing service, which must support and complement institutional goals. In an institution with an overall goal of developing a bone marrow transplant program, a nursing department goal might include developing nursing expertise in the care of bone marrow transplant patients. In the institution with goals directed toward manpower availability, the nursing department might identify specific goals aimed at retaining nursing personnel.

The astute manager of a nursing department must also be proactive in regard to the national issues facing nursing, community needs for nursing, and the needs within the institution itself. This manager would formulate goals to help the nursing department meet the challenges of care in the future, because the ultimate nursing department goal is quality client care.

Nursing Unit Goals

It is important that each employee understand the institutional and nursing department goals, because the group or unit goals develop from them. Each nurse should be able to contribute to the formation of unit goals in terms of philosophy of care, quality of care, and development of nursing expertise.

Helping to formulate the goals for your unit is important, because these goals can also represent your individual goals. Unit goals develop from the group as a whole and often include individual goals in the process. For example, you may have a particular interest in client teaching and hope to develop your own expertise in this area. If you assist in formulating goals for your unit that include the expansion and improvement of client teaching, you may thereby help to meet your own goals for professional growth. In this example, you might be able to work with a client teaching committee to develop standardized teaching protocols for commonly occurring needs on your unit.

Development and implementation of goals must be meaningful to the group if they are to be successful. The members of the group must feel that they are the originators of the unit goals and objectives. As a manager you should not set up goals and objectives independently for the unit. This would only result in your feeling frustrated and disappointed. You must give top priority to involving the staff in developing these goals. If you are the nurse manager, it is important to communicate institutional and nursing department goals as you plan with your staff so that you can help them understand the context in which they are planning.

In the real world of nursing practice, you will most often work with a team of professionals who all want quality client care. For this to occur the nurse manager must communicate clearly his or her understanding of the situation to those with whom the responsibility of the work is shared. Then together you can write goals so they can be understood.

The following example illustrates the importance of clearly agreeing on written goals and objectives. Driving home from work one day, a nurse could ponder the idea that the quality of nursing care plans written on the unit should be improved. The first casual thought was, "The care plans need to be better." How would that concept be translated into a meaningful goal with objectives?

This nurse needs to help others see this need and to write the goal to maximize the probability of achievement. Simply stating to the nursing staff, "The care plans need to be better," would not assure the achievement of the goal. What is the overall picture of what is desirable? Two possibilities for "better" care plans follow.

Goal: The client and/or client family will be involved in developing the plan of care.

Objectives
1. Initiate all nursing care plans with an interview of the client or the client's significant other.
2. Clearly record the client/family anticipated outcome of care in the Outcome Column of the care plan.
3. Chart once every 24 hours regarding the nursing care provided to meet the client/family expected outcome of care.

A "better" care plan could also look like this:

Goal: Use only North American Nursing Diagnosis Association (NANDA) nursing diagnoses on all care plans.

Objectives
1. Schedule all registered nurses to attend inservice class on the use of NANDA terminology.
2. Purchase 10 NANDA handbooks for use on the unit.

3. Establish a team of three RNs to evaluate care plans as to their use of nursing diagnosis and provide feedback to the staff.

The idea is that both goals will result in the care plans being better. However, all the staff nurses will not understand what is better unless the goal is written clearly, in a manner that reflects the concepts of the nurses on that unit. Objectives must be written with the specific behaviors in mind that are expected from the staff, from the client, or from whomever the objective is intended.

This idea of accurate communication should assist you in understanding why goals and objectives are important. The example of the two approaches to the better care plans should make it clear that a very general concept can look very different to different people and that clear and specific goals and objectives help everyone work together more effectively.

PERSONAL GOALS AND OBJECTIVES

Setting goals and implementing actions to achieve those goals is becoming increasingly important in health care today. A nurse who knows how to develop goals and achieve them is a valuable asset to the health care team. By examining your own individual, professional, and personal goals, you can determine the direction of your career in nursing. Family responsibilities and a desire for advanced and personal development all need to be thoughtfully examined and priorities must be set.

After determining your goals, the next step is to break them down into short-range and long-range goals. Then you should decide on the activities that will help achieve your goals. You should always try to be clear and concise in developing the action plan that will lead to goal attainment.

It is important to share your professional goals with those who can assist you in their attainment. An example of this is given by the new nurse who has the long-term goal of becoming a nurse administrator. By sharing this with the head nurse he or she might ask for some administrative assignments that would benefit the new nurse as well as relieve the head nurse of certain tasks. Asking for feedback and evaluation on your performance will assist you in determining if the goals you have set are realistic. Patience and flexibility are important attributes to develop as you move toward attainment of your goals.

Right now is a good time for you to think personally about goals and objectives. Where are *you* going and how will you know when you get there? This question could refer to either a personal or professional goal. What is your 6-month, 12-month, and 5-year plan? Even more pragmatically, what is your top priority for tomorrow? *Stop right now* and think about one of your goals. Can you see what it looks like as you work on it and what it will be when it is completed? Stop and really give one of your goals some thought. Ask yourself the following questions about your goal:

- Is it fuzzy? Or can you clearly see what it will look like when completed?
- Can you differentiate between the goal (the overall picture of what you want to achieve) and the objectives (the steps that will lead you to the goal)?

The goal will tell you "what it will look like when you get there" and the objectives should clarify how you will "get there!"

Relating Personal Goals to Unit and Institutional Goals

The reality of being a clinical nurse manager is that you often want to do more than is actually realistic. In addition, others, both above you and below you in the hierarchy, may expect or demand more than is actually possible. This "super nurse" syndrome can usually be managed by writing and sharing goals and objectives. This is an effective method of prioritizing the demands that are placed upon you as well as sharing a realistic picture of the workload with others.

For the nurse manager a Monday morning may bring with it:

- A commitment to finish the annual budget and submit it to your supervisor today, the deadline date for submission.
- Appointments with three employees to review their evaluations. You need approximately 45 minutes to finish the evaluation forms.
- The night nurse has fallen and twisted his ankle. He will not be in for the next three night shifts and there is no automatic coverage.
- An angry client family member just called to say he wanted to speak to the "nurse in charge right away." You expect him in about 10 minutes.

This is the type of stressful situation in which established goals may assist the nurse manager in determining priorities. Without examining the overall goals of the institution or unit managed by the nurse, there would be a feeling of concern if the manager stayed in his or her office and finished the annual budget and the performance evaluations rather than dealing with the staffing situation and/or the angry family member. However, the manager might delegate the replacement of the night nurse to someone experienced in that area, meet with the family member and the employees, and postpone working on the annual budget. This may seem like the logical sequence of planning; however, consider how that would change if the overall goal of the institution was written as follows:

Goal: "In the black" budgeting of the departments in this institution will be the primary method of evaluation and determination of future fund allocations.

Objectives
1. All budgets will be turned into the administrator on or before the due date.
2. Ninety-five percent of the middle management evaluation will be based on the effectiveness and timeliness of the budget.

This goal and set of objectives are unappealing, but an administrator who has written this "in the black" goal would certainly determine how the Monday morning nurse manager would set the priorities of the day. Do you notice how a different institutional goal changes the priority setting completely?

Goal: The use of interpersonal relationship skills with medical and nursing staff, clients, and families will be the primary focus of all charge nurses.

Objective
1. All client and family complaints will be dealt with personally by the charge nurse.
2. Personnel evaluations will be done in a one-on-one setting with each employee.
3. The charge nurse will communicate with each client once a shift.

Institutional goals are a great deal like the "better" care plan. No one knows if client/family involvement or the use of the NANDA list of diagnoses is the most important unless someone has shared the goal. Knowing that client/family involvement is a factor in how the administrator defines "better" care needs to be clearly stated in order to determine how to handle priorities.

Knowing the goals of the institution will determine the behaviors of the nurse. The goals of the overall organization can be reviewed before beginning employment, before accepting a promotion, and, if necessary, before planning a Monday morning priority list.

Consider the scenario of a nurse who graduated from a religiously based school of nursing that taught the nursing care philosophy of serving the sick as if the nurse were Christ in person. Once this nurse graduated, an opportunity occurred for employment as the evening charge nurse at a major medical center. With a great deal of first-job enthusiasm, the nurse began her new job. Try to imagine the reaction of the nurse when the hospital carefully listed its overall goals as teaching, research, and client care, in that order! Those goals were in direct conflict with the long-established goals of nursing care of the nurse. Eventually, her employment at that facility became impossible because of the personal conflict resulting from the two sets of goals.

You have been able to review some examples of what proactive institutional and nursing service organizations might be looking at in setting organizational goals. If you were a nurse employed in such a proactive setting, how would your professional goals and objectives mesh with what was happening? Some would not find enough emphasis on educational advancement; others would consider that there was too much effort going into trying to determine "everyone's" opinion. Someone would be certain to notice that very little had been listed that absolutely and directly impacted on the quality of care given at the bedside. Some of that content is inferred, but little of it is directly noted and would be of concern to some nurses.

Now take a minute and go back to the goals and objectives you thought about earlier in this chapter that were directed to your profession. Think over what you visualized as your professional goals and determine in what type of institutional setting you would work best, have your skills and knowledge most utilized, and generally be able to meet your goals while employed there.

A PROBLEM RELATED TO GOAL SETTING

When thinking of goals and objectives on a personal level and relating them to your career, you need to match your goals with those of nursing service, which should also match those of the institution. One common problem found in many institutions, especially those without clear-cut operational goals, is *goal displacement*.

Goal Displacement

Goal displacement means that a unit in the institution (such as a nursing unit) pursues its own narrowly defined goals rather than the overall goals of the institution. Sometimes goal displacement manifests itself with extreme bureaucratic behavior (Sullivan & Decker, 1988). This rule-driven behavior does not allow for flexibility, individuality, or diversity of nursing practice. It could be the charge nurse who will not tolerate allowing a Vietnamese family to remain with their ill family member 24 hours a day or the staff nurse who will not wait 10 minutes for report on a busy day. When an entire unit is experiencing goal displacement, the unit may look very efficient, because all the rules are being followed, but compassion seems to be missing. There is little tolerance for mistakes made by other departments or units and, therefore, minimal willingness to resolve problems inside and outside of the unit.

This attention to rules rather than process or outcome of behavior does not allow individual input and contribution, flexibility of problem solving, or development of meaningful goals and objectives. This occurs most often in bureaucratic organizations and/or when the goals of the institution are general and ambiguous. The pursuit of a unit's own goals almost naturally occurs when the institution's goals are so unclear that they cannot be followed effectively. If several units and/or departments are experiencing goal displacement, the environment is ready for conflict. This type of distress occurs because of the competition for scarce resources, lack of focus as an institution, and incompatible goals.

Resolving Problems Related to Goals

Although the nurse manager frequently does not have direct responsibility for resolving an institution-wide conflict, it is important to understand the nature of the conflict as well as some of the techniques for conflict resolution. As a registered nurse, you may be asked to participate in planning conferences where institutional or unit goals are rewritten because of a conflict. The most frequent need is that of changing or clarifying goals. The strength of the institutional goals must be obvious to each unit for change to be effective.

Another common method of resolving conflict of this type is the development of a superordinate goal. A *superordinate goal* is a goal of high appeal value for the groups involved but whose attainment is beyond the resources and efforts of any one group.

Research by Hungler and Stern (1976) indicates that superordinate goals can be effective in resolving conflict between groups even though some of the underlying causes of the conflict may remain unchanged. A superordinate goal is exemplified by a facility desiring accreditation or survey approval for Medicare and Medicaid. All employees will realize that their employment depends on achieving the approval being sought by the facility's administration, because the survival of the institution is at stake. Therefore, this is a superordinate goal. Rather than departments fighting fiercely for limited dollars for development of their department alone, all departments will generally work together to meet the requirements of the survey or accreditation, so that every department will survive. Generally, after the superordinate goal is no longer in place, the individual departments resume their conflict over scarce resources if that conflict existed before the superordinate goal surfaced.

In health care facilities there is an automatic superordinate goal: quality client care. However, if units in the facility are involved in their own goal displacement, it may take someone with authority on the administrative level to remind them of that superordinate goal. Whenever conflict surfaces for you, the nurse, the superordinate goal of client care is one concept to keep clearly in mind. You may need to evaluate the goals of the unit as well as those of the individual nurses and if necessary encourage a restandardization of those goals toward the superordinate goal.

INCREASING NURSING POWER IN THE INSTITUTION

When the nurse has a clear concept of personal, unit, and institutional goals and objectives, he or she has an immediate reward: power. Nursing is an integral part of management and must participate within the group and carry out management decisions. The power base for the responsibility of management is clarified when goals are strengthened and realistic objectives are defined for achieving those goals. The power of the individual nurse and the nursing service department increases when there is goal congruency among all levels of management. Do you remember the nurse who could not support the goals of the medical center? Because of the incompatibility of the institution's goals and those of the nurse, not only was she frustrated enough to leave her position, but while there, she was unable to support the goals of the institution.

Personal Power

Prior to accepting any position, you should thoroughly discuss institutional and personal philosophies of nursing with the potential employer. After discussing philosophies you should discuss your professional goals. When a nurse can line up personal goals with those of the institution, so that they are compatible, the work of the institution is done more effectively and the power of the nurse is increased greatly.

Nursing Responsibilities

The real power in nursing occurs when the quality of care delivered at the bedside can be planned and implemented by the registered nurse. This is where the nurse, in whatever position—manager, clinician, or educator—should want to make an impact. A reasonable method of achieving that impact is through goal-directed client care based on nursing diagnosis.

If the profession of nursing cannot deliver the overall product of the profession, nursing care, it is not significant how well other professional behaviors (*i.e.,* education, research, management) are performed. The measurement of success is at the side of the client, and that success is strongly enhanced when the care is planned and delivered by a goal-oriented professional working in an environment where personal goals match institutional goals and objectives.

THE EVALUATION PROCESS

The final process for looking at goal effectiveness is that of evaluation. Effectiveness, as a managerial concept, is the satisfactory achievement of one's goals. In nursing there are several measures of effectiveness:

1. Quality control (quality assurance) tools and systems measure the statistical effectiveness of nursing care in reaching defined or selected client care goals.
2. Performance appraisal tools and systems measure the effectiveness of performance of the individual worker.
3. The evaluation component of the nursing care plan determines the success or failure in individual client care.
4. External review standards, such as the Joint Commission on Accreditation of Health Care Organization, and internally derived standards serve to supply criteria for evaluating a nursing unit's operational effectiveness (Stevens, 1980).

After carefully writing and implementing the goals and objectives of the nursing unit, the process of evaluation begins by means of one of the processes listed. It is important to remember that all goals should be evaluated and that the evaluation is necessary to measure failure or success.

Evaluation serves several purposes. It measures the effectiveness with which the members of the unit staff achieve their goals and objectives. It also serves as a guide for change and improvement. The more specific you are in writing the goals and objectives, the easier the evaluation process will be to carry out.

Evaluation tools and standards need to flow from clearly stated goals and objectives. After goals are developed at the institution, unit, or personal level, the objectives to meet the goals must be written in measurable terms. If the objective is not written in measurable terms, the evaluation process becomes subjective and ambiguous. At the beginning of evaluation for any program, the objectives must be scrutinized carefully for clarity and conciseness.

Developing Evaluation Tools

Evaluation may be carried out by various methods: direct observation of individual performance, paper-and-pencil tests of knowledge, and/or surveys of client satisfaction. The method you choose to use for evaluation will depend on what you are going to evaluate and the plan you have for utilizing the evaluative information. Of course, this would be predetermined by the goals you have set for yourself, the unit, or the institution. When developing forms that will evaluate goals and objectives, several suggestions will facilitate the process (Rowland & Rowland, 1985):

1. Express only one idea with each item evaluated.
2. Use words the evaluator will understand.
3. Have evaluators evaluate what they observe, not what is inferred.
4. Avoid double negatives.
5. Express thoughts clearly and simply.
6. Keep statements internally consistent.
7. Avoid universal statements.
8. Concentrate on the present.
9. Avoid vague concepts.

These guidelines will help you prepare forms that accurately evaluate your goals and objectives. Not only should your evaluations be prepared using these guidelines, but this type of preparation assumes a written evaluation that is kept on file for reference.

In analyzing the evaluation material, you will need to refer back to your objectives. The process calls for scrutiny of behaviors in staff, clients, and others that will indicate the objectives have been met. (See Chapter 10 for a discussion of evaluating individual performance.)

Utilization of Evaluation

The value of this evaluation process is enhanced when the results are shared with appropriate members of the health care team. This team effort at analyzing the evaluation of a specific set of goals and objectives will give credibility to both the process and results of the goal-setting procedure. The primary purpose of evaluation is to determine the need for change. The nurse will use the results in the evaluation process to make the changes needed.

QUALITY ASSURANCE

A current concern in all of health care is assuring that quality of care remains high.

> We have granted the health professions access to the most secret and sensitive places in ourselves, and entrusted to them matters that touch on our well-being, happiness and survival. In return we have expected the professions to govern themselves so strictly that we need have no fear of exploitation or incompetence. The object of quality assessment is to determine how successful they have been in doing so; and the purpose of quality monitoring

is to exercise constant surveillance so that departure from standards can be detected early and corrected [Donabedian, 1978].

The concept of quality assurance (QA) tools and systems is a valid one within the discussion of goals and objectives in nursing management. QA calls for concrete, quantitative written standards and is defined in relationship to nursing standards of care and legal responsibilities. As the essence of professional nursing, quality assurance is the defining of nursing practice through well-written nursing standards and the use of those standards as a basis for evaluation and improvement of client care (Marker, 1988). The use of well-written standards as nursing goals and objectives serves to enhance the quality assurance process.

As planning is carried out for quality assurance in the institution, it is essential that those individuals responsible for implementing the quality assurance program be involved in the process. Understanding of, confidence in, and commitment to goal achievement result from the participation of nursing staff in developing the goals and objectives for the quality assurance program. A successful program is never planned, implemented, and evaluated in a vacuum. Successful planning for quality assurance begins at the individual unit level and with the staff nurse who can effectively use the goal-setting process.

History of Quality Assurance Programs

In October 1972, the Ninety-second Congress passed Public Health Law 92-603, an amendment to the Social Security Act that mandated the establishment of Professional Standards Review Organizations (PSRO) to review the quality and cost of care received by Medicare, Medicaid, and Maternal Child Health programs (Marriner-Tomey, 1988). Health facilities were challenged to develop quality control programs by 1976 or else have the government do it for them. As a consequence, quality assurance programs have received considerable attention over the past decade from the government as well as from private health care facilities, to the point that PSROs have been replaced by professional review organizations (PROs) and that every accredited health care facility supports a quality assurance program.

As part of its widely publicized 1989 Agenda for Change, the Joint Commission for Accreditation of Health Care Organizations developed a new accrediting process that included three major initiatives: (1) a substantial revision of the accreditation manual; (2) a uniform set of indicators of patient care quality for specific clinical and organizational units to be collected from each hospital and incorporated into a national data base; and (3) a modification of survey and accreditation methods (American Hospital Association, 1989). These changes clearly represent a far-reaching effort by the Joint Commission to expand upon its current quality assurance requirement, the implications of which will continue to evolve over the next several years. Independent of additional requirements that may be defined by the Agenda for Change, the Joint Commission has specified a model for quality assurance that accredited health care facilities are now required to have.

The 1989 Accreditation Manual for Hospitals "Quality Assurance" chapter states that for each facility "there is an ongoing quality assurance program designed to objectively and systematically monitor and evaluate the quality and appropriateness of patient care, pursue opportunities to improve patient care and resolve identified problems." The role of the nurse in this process is critical. Any patient care review is only as good as its measurement criteria, and the criteria are only as appropriate as the standards from which they come. Staff nurses are involved in writing standards and reviewing criteria.

Developing criteria is not distasteful; rather, it is a professional activity accomplished through group process and priority setting. Criteria are purposefully selected variables of care that, if met, reflect compliance to a standard and, if not met, reflect noncompliance. This approach to thinking should resemble the process of setting goals and objectives. Determining quality effectiveness and efficiency depends on sound definitions and measurable components of quality, or, more specifically, the goal-setting process. Without cognitively processed and well-written goals and objectives, quality assurance programs do not have a framework within which to work.

Framework of Quality Assurance Programs

The goal-oriented framework of quality assurance includes three areas: structure, process, and outcome. The *structure approach* focuses on the delivery system where nursing care is implemented. Quality assurance committee members evaluate policies, procedures, job descriptions, orientation schedules, inservice schedules, and other types of organizational factors. The *process approach* examines what the employee does while delivering client care. The *outcome approach* examines the results of the care administered to the client and evaluates to see if the goals were reached by considering clinical manifestations, client knowledge, and the client's self-care. The results or data gathered from any of these processes and the process itself are called the *audit*.

Quality Assurance Audits

Audits for quality assurance can be concurrent or retrospective. *Concurrent reviews* or audits evaluate care as it is being administered and may include observation of the staff, inspection of the client, open-chart

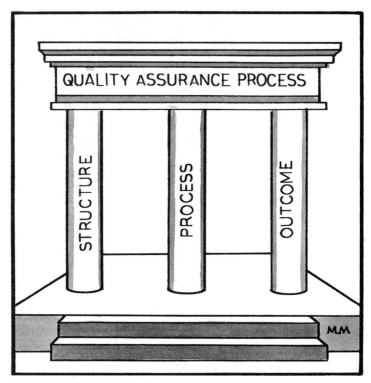

The goal-oriented framework of quality assurance includes structure, process, and outcome.

auditing, staff and client interviews, and group conferences that include participation from the client, family, and staff. *Retrospective reviews* audit care after it has been delivered; these reviews are done through study of client charts or care plans after the client has been discharged, postcare questionnaires, and/or client interviews (Marriner-Tomey, 1988).

Nursing and Quality Assurance

The individual responsibility of the bedside or managerial nurse in the quality assurance process is a critical one. The American Nurses' Association (ANA) has suggested that Standards of Nursing Practice set forth by the ANA Divisions of Practice can be applied in any clinical situation and therefore can serve as a professional nursing model for quality assurance.

Quality assurance is a professional responsibility. The days of a 3-day postoperative period for a hernia repair are gone. In their stead is the responsibility of teaching, treating according to human response patterns, and nurturing the client to his best possible health in a much more limited span of time. It is expected that this client will not only be treated more quickly but *better* (does this remind you of the "better" nursing care plans at the beginning of the chapter?), and by means of a process that can be concretely evaluated according to written goals.

QA presents opportunities for nurses to have a voice in the control of nursing practice. The procedure is for the nursing service administrator to be responsible for initiation and maintenance of a nursing QA program. The methods used should have been predetermined by the nursing staff and may include established standards of care, measurement of actual practice against standards and criteria, and evaluation of results. These standards are set by means of the work done in committees. Some committees may be nursing only; others may be interdisciplinary. The input from *you,* the nurse, is critical to assurance of quality to clients. It is then the nursing manager's responsibility to reinforce strengths and to correct deficiencies in nursing service (Douglass, 1988).

Utilization of Quality Assurance Evaluation

The utilization of the evaluation data is as important as gathering the data. The quality assurance committee must determine the level of expected performance below which it will take corrective action. The nursing staff should know what criteria are being used to evaluate the quality of care and should have an opportunity to review reports of audits. The committee formally identifies performance discrepancies and completes an analysis of the problem. Once the problem is identified, the committee should recommend corrective measures. Then the corrective action, recommended time schedule for completion, and person designated as responsible for followthrough are documented and shared with appropriate persons. A reaudit determines if the corrective action was implemented successfully and the stated goals met. It is also important to share with staff favorable audits and evidence of improvement in care.

The actual utilization of QA or evaluation data is critical. Its importance can be underlined with the following stories. After having a total hip replacement done on the wrong hip (a situation that left the client in a wheelchair), the large, metropolitan hospital where this happened instituted an additional check in a system that already had five different checks to prevent this type of error. The morning of surgery the client and/or his family mark with a permanent marker the hip or other joint that is to have the surgery. This is a simple solution to a serious problem.

A lack of compliance with a basic safeguard of care caused another hazard for a client. While in the field on an emergency, a Life Flight nurse inserted an endotracheal tube without wearing gloves. The first point of concern is generally for the nurse. However, in this particular situation it was the client who developed a *Staphylococcus aureus* in her lungs because of the less than hygienic hands of the nurse. The client became septic and spent 5 days in ICU being treated for that infection. This problem was identified through a QA audit. A change in procedure could then be initiated.

Compliance with and management of quality assurance for all clients will result in exactly what it should—an assurance of quality care to those dependent on the professional nurse for that care.

SUMMARY

Clearly stated goals and objectives provide guidance and direction in the delivery of quality client care. The goals and objectives of the institution and the nursing department will provide guidance for the nurse manager in developing the goals and objectives for the individual nursing units. Personal career goals of the nurse need to fit within the institutional and nursing unit goals for maximizing client care. Evaluation of client care becomes more effective when goals and objectives have been closely stated in measurable terms. Objectives for meeting these goals are written as the plan of care and thus can be evaluated in an objective manner.

Quality assurance assists in the delivery of quality nursing care by defining nursing practice through written standards against which care is evaluated. The nurse manager and staff utilize all of these concepts in planning and implementing safe, quality nursing care.

Study Questions/Activities

1. Write your personal philosophy of nursing.
2. Compare and contrast your philosophy of nursing with that of a nursing service department. If possible, the nursing department should be from a facility where you work or plan to work.
3. Locate the quality assurance manual and standards of care for a nursing unit. Review that material and follow one standard of care on a client to determine how the process works.
4. Write a personal goal as discussed in the chapter, with one goal and three objectives.
5. Write your professional goals as discussed in the chapter, with one goal and three objectives. Add to that information a statement regarding your 5-year and 10-year professional plans.

6. Discuss with a practicing registered nurse the concept of goal displacement on a unit and how resolution of that conflict can be achieved.
7. Review the unit goals of a clinical area as to how the goals are written and discuss their practicality for you as a nurse.
8. "Power in nursing is best demonstrated at the bedside." Discuss how this concept affects your power base and the manner in which you would like to develop it.
9. Discuss the difference between concurrent and retrospective quality assurance reviews.

REFERENCES

American Hospital Association Division of Quality Control Management (1989). *Technical briefing: The joint commission quality assurance model.* Kansas City, Kan.: The Association.

Douglass, L.M. (1988). *The effective nurse manager,* 3rd ed. St. Louis: C.V. Mosby.

Marker, C.G. (1988). Practical tools for quality assurance: Criteria development sheet and data retrieval form. *Journal of Nursing Quality Assurance, 2*(2), 43–54.

Marriner-Tomey, A. (1988). *Guide to nursing management,* 3rd ed. St. Louis: C.V. Mosby.

Rowland, H.S., & Rowland, B. (1985). *Nursing administration handbook,* 2nd ed. Rockville, Md.: Aspen Publication.

Stevens, B.J. (1980). *The nurse as executive,* 2nd ed. Wakefield, Mass.: Nursing Resources, Inc.

Sullivan, E.J., & Decker, P.J. (1985). *Effective management in nursing.* Reading, Mass.: Addison-Wesley.

SUGGESTIONS FOR FURTHER READING

Carlson, C., Davis, K., Marks, S., & Toney, J. (1987). An effective management tool for nursing. *AD Nurse, 19*(5), 86–93.

Carpenito, L. (1987). *Nursing diagnosis: Application to clinical practice,* 2nd ed. Philadelphia: J.B. Lippincott.

Donabedian, A. (1984). Quality, cost, and cost containment. *Nursing Outlook, 32*(3), 56–59.

Hampshire, G. (1983). Defining goals . . . the basis of systematic care. *Nursing-Times, 20*(3), 16–22.

Hegge, M.J. (1986). A fresh approach to group goal setting: The three-way rotation nominal group technique. *Journal of Nursing Staff Development, 2*(1), 52–54.

Linc, L.G. (1987). Institutional goal analysis: An approach to program evaluation. *Journal of Nursing Education, 26*(4), 36.

Mager, R.F. (1962). *Preparing instructional objectives.* Belmont, Calif.: Fearon Publishers.

Ride, T. (1984). Going for goal . . . why it is important for nurses to have goals. *Nursing-Mirror, 14*(9), 26–27.

Strasen, L. (1988). Nursing-management, strategic planning: Nursing process how-to's. *AD Nurse, 2*(1), 18–21.

Trexler, B.J. (1987). Nursing department purpose, philosophy, and objectives: Their use and effectiveness. *Journal of Nursing Administration, 11*(3), 42–47.

Vogelberger, M.L. (1986). A new approach to the care plan problem. *Journal of Nursing Staff Development, 12*(3), 120–125.

Understanding Power

4

Objectives

After completing this chapter, you should be able to

1. *Write a personal definition of power.*
2. *Discuss resources for power within yourself.*
3. *Define seven types of power.*
4. *Identify methods for increasing your personal power.*
5. *Discuss ways of using power effectively.*
6. *List possible consequences of the use of power.*

The term *power* evokes many different feelings. The power of a hurricane or an earthquake is frightening and destructive. The power of electricity provides heat when it is cold, coolness when it is hot, and feelings of comfort. The power of a gasoline engine represents freedom to go when and where we wish. When we describe a person as powerful, we also evoke feelings. Sometimes we fear that a person will use power coercively against us or others. We may feel in awe of the power of an individual who is able to accomplish significant tasks. We may feel envy for the advantages we see accruing to the powerful person.

Similarly, people have many different attitudes about power. Some seek it diligently; others avoid it at all costs. Still others have never given it any thought in regard to themselves. But what exactly is power and how does it relate to your role as a nurse?

DEFINITIONS OF POWER

Power has many different meanings. The dictionary defines it as "the ability to do or act; the capability of doing or accomplishing something" (*Random House Dictionary*, 1985). This definition can be applied to many different situations. Engines, animals, and people can all possess power under this definition. A person has power when he or she can act or accomplish something. In nursing, the clearest example using this definition of *power* might be provided by the patient who, because of a cervical spinal cord injury, cannot move any part of his or her body. This person lacks the power to do any task.

In the psychological and sociological literature, power is used to describe an ability to control and influence others (Dahl, 1957; Bierstedt, 1950; Hesse-Biber & Williamson, 1984). The view of power as control is also seen in the business literature (Petrellis, 1985). In nursing we might identify the director of nursing service as powerful because he or she has ultimate control over who will be assigned as unit managers and whether they will remain in those positions. Josefowitz states, "We take power to mean forcefulness—the ability or official capacity to exercise control" (1980). Power in business is treated as essential to promotion and success. In nursing, the control of others might occur when the charge nurse makes patient assignments and determines who is to do the necessary tasks for the shift. A nurse who does this well might be more likely to be selected for promotion to assistant nurse manager for the unit.

Claus and Bailey (1977) pointed out that "power is a pyramid having elements of ability, based on strength, willingness based on energy, and action that yields results." These authors discuss power as important for individuals who have goals they want to accomplish. Without ability you will not be able to do what you wish. Without strength you cannot carry out desired tasks, and without the willingness to act you may never begin.

For our purposes we will return to the simple dictionary definition, "the capability of doing or accomplishing something." The powerful person, then, is one who is able to accomplish desired ends. These ends may be accomplished through personal actions or through the actions of others, but the true sign of power is accomplishment.

Power from this standpoint is very important to nurses and nursing. Nursing has much to contribute to health care, and individual nurses need to be effective in a wide variety of settings. There are many different forces acting upon the health care system, some of which do not share nursing's values for the autonomy and integrity of the person and health as a primary goal. Without power nurses find themselves thwarted in their efforts and unable to accomplish what they see as important. Understanding, acquiring, and using power will help nurses to move forward in the achievement of their goals for clients and for the system.

QUANTIFYING POWER

Power as presented in all the different definitions is not a static phenomenon, but rather a varied and changing concept. We all see that power differs between individuals and within the same individual at different times. It is possible to speak of having no power or great power. This leads to the conclusion that power can be measured. In some instances researchers have attempted to measure exact quantities of power (Stevenson, 1982).

As we look at quantities of power, another question arises: Is the quantity of power in any given situation subject to some limit; is there a specific quantity of power in a given situation and no more? If power in any situation is limited, then those who wish to exercise more power must obtain it from someone else who possesses it. This may lead to conflict. Concern regarding this kind of conflict is one reason some people do not wish to seek power.

On the other hand, if we believe that power is not limited in any situation but that it can expand and contract in total quantity, then one individual can increase power without decreasing the power of someone else. This means that seeking power does not necessarily bring you into conflict with others. If you look back at the definition and regard power as being able to accomplish what you wish to accomplish, then it is possible for more than one person to hold power. This does not mean that conflict will always be avoidable. If two people with power want opposing things, if they have differing goals, then they will find themselves in conflict. (Chapter 11 discusses approaches to managing conflict constructively.)

POWER AND NURSING

Value judgments about power are found widely in the literature. Lippitt (1983) states that one has increased feelings of self-worth, respect of others, shared hopes, and mutual support when one wields power. On the other hand, Tannenbaum and Cook (1974) state that there is a common distaste for the idea of power, which they relate to the unpleasant connotation of control in a democratic society. This may be one reason some nurses are reluctant to seek and develop power openly. Additionally, nursing is a caring profession, focused on others, and those in nursing generally have a strong commitment to a nurturing role. It is not uncommon for nurses to regard the pursuit of power as inappropriate to the nurse, because they see it as controlling rather than as supporting others.

Those who avoid power or reject its use often do so because they consider it to be bad. Rollo May (1972) wrote that power is the birthright of all human beings, that power and love are interrelated. We must have power within ourselves to love one another. He further says that the pseudoinnocence that rejects power is often a shield from reality and growth, a shield that protects us from new awareness of ourselves and others and from identifying with the suffering and joys of each person.

In the world of modern health care it is increasingly apparent that nurses need to affect the way that health care is delivered, the priorities that are set within health care, and the kind of care received by clients. Because of their educational backgrounds, their continued close relationships with individual clients, and their overall commitment to health, nurses have special knowledge and skills to bring to any decision-making process. Nursing as a whole is moving into this new role in health care.

In any system those with more power are more likely to accomplish the goals they see as important. Therefore, if nurses are to reach their potential and support the health care needs of clients, they need to look at their power in the health care system.

TYPES OF POWER

French and Raven (1965) identified five types of power based on the source: legitimate, referent, reward, expert, and coercive. These five types can be seen in many different settings.

Legitimate power, often termed *authority,* arises from an organizational structure and policies that place control in specific positions within that organization. In general, whoever holds the position has the same amount of authority. This authority may include making decisions on behalf of the organization, acquiring or controlling information, having access to people of higher status or power, and control of the human and material resources of the organization. The person who holds legitimate power is usually given a title to indicate the authority that has been delegated.

The head nurse or the unit manager has legitimate power associated with the responsibility for a patient care unit. The head nurse may develop and control the budget at the unit level, hire staff, and meet regularly with those at the next higher level in the organization. He or she can require that an individual alter behavior within the job. As a charge nurse on the evening shift you would have authority delegated to you by the head nurse. You might have the authority to make all patient assignments and determine who will float to another unit for the evening.

Referent power is control that derives its base in personal characteristics of a powerful person. The term *charisma* has also been used to describe referent power. This is the type of power often seen in political figures. Those who exhibit charisma are able to garner votes and be reelected. In the hospital setting, a very popular and outgoing nurse may influence decisions in ways that do not reflect any official position in the organization.

Another aspect of referent power is appearing to be a powerful person. Behavior that says, "I am confident, sure of myself, and in charge," tends to encourage others to ascribe power to the individual. Those with referent power remain calm in crisis, control their emotional responses, and act with firm determination. This type of behavior was historically

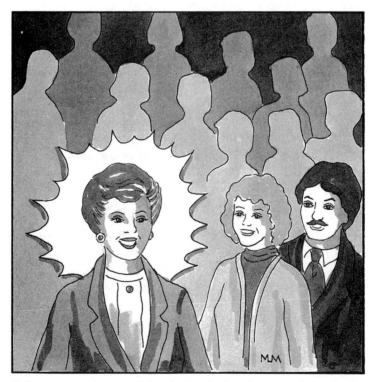

Referent power is control that derives its base in personal characteristics of a powerful person.

seen as "male" behavior, and some women have had difficulty reconciling their desire to appear powerful with their concern about not appearing unfeminine.

Manner of dress has also been associated with referent power. Business people speak of "power dressing" or wearing a "power suit." Much of this is based on the research of John Molloy, who has examined the responses of people to various forms of dress (Molloy, 1988). His conclusions were that most people associate certain types of clothing with power. The majority of powerful people in business environments dress conservatively and avoid extremes of fashion. Their clothing is of good quality and always well cared for. They present themselves as businesslike and avoid a social appearance in the business environment. Others who adopt this appearance are regarded as possessing power and status. Although first impressions may not persist, positive first impressions provide an added advantage to the individual.

Reward power helps people exert control through providing reward or the promise of reward to others. Although the person with legitimate power may control rewards, many other people also control rewards in any given environment. A client controls the rewards associated with positive feedback for the care that you provide. You control rewards of praise and recognition given to coworkers.

Expert power helps individuals attain control through the possession of special knowledge, skill, or ability. Experts are able to accomplish their ends because others recognize their knowledge and ability and turn to them for guidance. When experts give an opinion it has more weight in any decision than an opinion given by someone without expert knowledge. A clinical nursing specialist may not have direct authority over the behavior of individual nurses and therefore may not evaluate or promote these nurses. Nevertheless, the clinical nursing specialist is able to alter the manner in which care is delivered on a nursing unit by providing information and resources and suggesting appropriate changes in care.

Coercive power allows people to attain control through fear, threat, or coercion. The power of some authoritarian leaders is coercive. They control through fear of loss of job or of punishment, such as undesirable assignments or shifts. Your first response may be that coercive power is inherently inappropriate. However, some situations may require coercion. The law exercises coercive power to maintain safety for citizens. In a hospital setting, coercion is sometimes used to solve problems that involve potential danger to clients. For example, if a nurse is discovered to be abusing drugs, the threat of loss of license, job, and ability to support herself may force her into an approved treatment and monitoring program. Although there may be philosophical support for self-direction in obtaining help, the safety of clients is so important that it must be the first consideration; therefore, coercion may be used when other avenues are unsuccessful.

In addition to these five basic sources of power, Hersey, Blanchard, and Natemeyer (1979) have added two other sources of power, connection power and knowledge power (see the accompanying display).

Connection power is control that is derived from a coalition of individuals working together or from the perception by others that an individual has connections with powerful persons or groups. The traditional stories of an individual having power in the workplace by marrying into the boss's family are outgrowths of the common recognition of connection power. But connection power is very important to nurses. Nursing is the single largest health care occupation. The force of all nurses working together could be phenomenal. Even within a patient care unit a group of nurses working cohesively toward a single goal will produce results. In a climate in which there is a shortage of nurses, this connectional power of nurses can be very strong. Nurses are negotiating contracts that recognize their expertise and value to the system. They are chairing important committees and gaining greater input into decision-making processes.

Information power occurs when a person controls information that is needed or could be used by others. This is not the same as expert power, which is specialized knowledge or expertise. Information that provides power may be knowledge of the institution's budget and income. Those without access to actual numbers may be stopped by a statement such as, "That is too expensive." They have no information with which to judge whether the organization's spending priorities are acceptable. The long-term care administrator who tells the nursing director that there is no money for additional patient care linen and then spends money left at the end of the fiscal year on redecorating offices has used knowledge power to

---

Types of Power

- *Legitimate power:* power through official authority from the organization
- *Referent power:* power through charisma and personal characteristics
- *Reward power:* power through providing rewards or promise of reward to others
- *Expert power:* power through possession of special knowledge, skill or ability
- *Coercive power:* power through fear, threat or coercion
- *Connection power:* power from coalition of individuals working together
- *Information power:* power from controlling or possessing information needed by others in the organization

his or her own ends. By not sharing in knowledge of the budget figures, others have no basis on which to criticize decisions that are made. It is not that the information is difficult or requires an expert to understand but that the information is necessary to enable others to affect the decisions that are made.

Information power may also be found in the person who has access to many different communication channels within an organization. Positions where this occurs as a structured part of the job are powerful ones. The person who knows what is happening in many different parts of an organization, what plans exist for the future, and what difficulties are being encountered has a greater opportunity to act effectively.

RESOURCES FOR DEVELOPING POWER

Various personal and material resources are necessary to develop power effectively. Personal resources include both physical and psychological ones. You must have energy. Without it you are powerless. Material resources may come from within the organization, but where and how they are used may vary greatly.

Physical Resources

Physical resources for power are the strengths you bring to each day's tasks. Health that provides energy and enthusiasm for activity is the base for the ability to act effectively. Nurses who recommend healthful living patterns, including diet, exercise, rest, and relaxation, to clients should incorporate those patterns into their own lives. Although some are successful in spite of the lack of physical health, the better your general health state, the easier it will be to become more powerful. Claus and Bailey (1977) state that individuals with power create positive vibrations that transmit mental, physical, and psychological energy.

Psychological Resources

The need for psychological resources for power is also apparent. The ability of the psychological system to affect work done over time may result in either more or less work than a person is capable of doing. This aspect of power is sometimes referred to as motivational power. Although some aspects of motivational power are within the awareness of the individual, many factors that affect this are outside of awareness. Motivation may be affected by self-esteem, interest, and the perceived value of the outcome. (Chapter 8 discusses motivation in greater detail.)

To achieve power you must develop a strong self-concept. Without a positive value of yourself and your abilities, others will not come to view you as competent and resourceful. Remember all you have learned in your psychology and psychosocial nursing courses about helping clients to develop self-esteem. This is equally important for you.

In addition to developing self-esteem you must have a clear awareness of your strengths and limitations. All of us have areas in which we do better. If we view these realistically, we can build on the strengths, use them creatively to offset areas in which we are not as strong. Limitations may be more constructively viewed as areas in which growth is needed. You can grow and change, altering those aspects of yourself that you see as needing development.

Another important point for those who would develop their personal power is maintaining a positive, forward outlook on the current situation. This does not imply that you ignore problems and difficulties but that you choose to view them as challenges to be overcome. When mistakes are made, you can look for solutions and directions for growth rather than for someone to blame.

This brings us to the final attribute that is important to developing power. That is problem-solving and decision making. Those who demonstrate power are also those who are creative problem solvers and

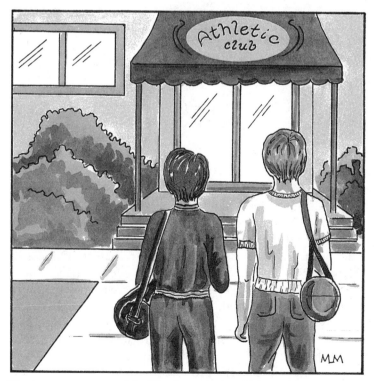

The better your general health, the easier it will be to become more powerful.

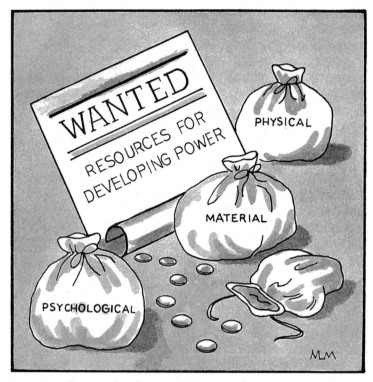

A variety of personal and material resources are necessary to develop power effectively.

effective decision makers. (Chapter 6 discusses approaches to effective decision making in greater detail.)

Material Resources

Material resources needed for the exercise of power may include money or objects. Without material resources some actions just are not possible. Even when material resources are available, if you do not control their use, then you lack this resource for your own action. Much power in our society derives from the control of material resources. On a state and national level, legislative bodies have power because they control the disbursement of the tax resources. In a health care agency the sources of payment (Medicare, Medicaid, insurance companies) exert control by determining what they will pay and in what circumstances they will pay. A hospital may find that maintaining a solid financial position depends on the surgeries that one group of surgeons brings to the hospital. This gives that group of surgeons power in the setting.

Nurses who control supplies, secretarial services, and copying facilities have a potential for power in an organization that is not possible for those who do not have these material resources. Those with authority in regard to the budget and spending have an important source of power. Others in the setting often identify powerful people by the external material resources that they can see controlled by an individual. An awareness of the need for material resources and where these are controlled is an essential base for developing power.

INCREASING YOUR POWER

Based on the preceding discussion, you can probably identify for yourself many ways in which you may increase your own power. Increasing your personal bases of power through improving health, energy, and self-esteem will enable you to act more effectively. You can examine your motivation and identify ways to increase it. As you work on personal growth, you can maintain a positive attitude and increase your own problem-solving and decision-making skills. Identify where in the organization material resources are controlled and how you may affect their use and allocation.

You may also increase your own power by attending to the specific types of power outlined. Legitimate power is increased by seeking a promotion or position of greater authority in an organization. Many people think that referent power is an inborn trait and not something one can develop. However, consider how politicians work to increase referent power through the way they dress, the way they treat people, and the publicity they choose. You will not be spending thousands on remaking your image, but you can change your image in some ways. Does the way you dress convey the image of someone who is responsible and in control? A confident attitude and an outgoing approach to others are other ways that can help increase your referent power.

Reward power is perhaps the type of power most readily increased. Rewards of salary and position are controlled by the official organization, but rewards of recognition and praise may be used by anyone. Do you recognize and commend others for a job well done or a difficult situation handled with poise and discretion? All too often we simply accept these examples of expertise from other nurses without comment rather than speaking up in commendation.

Expert power can be increased through continuing education, through inservice classes, and through independent reading and study. Many states require continuing education for nurses, but even in those that do not, individual nurses must take responsibility for their own education. As you gain in expertise you will be more able to affect the care setting in which you work.

Connection power is an area that nurses neglected for many years but one that they are increasingly recognizing as a valuable source of power. Nurses working together have organized practice committees in hospitals that have been able to alter policies and procedures and outcomes of patient care. Nurses working with others have supported the development of services for special client populations such as the homebound elderly and high-risk neonates. Through coalitions they have helped to raise public awareness of a variety of health concerns. Connection power will continue to be a growing resource for nurses in the future.

Knowledge power is an area that nurses often have not recognized as important to their own functioning. Gaining access to budgeting figures, planning details, and projections for growth will help nurses act more effectively. Where is the community growing, what areas of health care are showing the most demand, in what direction is the institution planning to move? These are all important questions that will provide nurses with a solid foundation.

There may even be times that you will need to use coercive power. An understanding of the legal requirements of your license may necessitate that you use this type of power on rare occasions. In some states nurses are required to report certain deficiencies in practice, such as client abuse that they observe. They may be in danger of losing their own license if they see such behavior and do not report it. You need a clear understanding of your own licensure law to understand the level of coercive power that is directed toward nurses and that you can use in selected instances.

USING POWER

Petrellis (1985) advises that the best use of power translates into getting things done through working effectively with others. He suggests that others are most likely to be cooperative and work with you when they see that they will gain from working with you. Part of what you must do is to recognize that you have a lot to give to others, including action, ideas, listening, promise of team effort, enthusiasm, encouragement, emotional support, acceptance, empathy, and appreciation of the other's abilities.

Nursing is enacted through interpersonal processes. Your relationships with colleagues, clients, families, and others in the health care field are fundamental to your accomplishments. From the beginning of your nursing education you were taught elements of effective interpersonal communication. These are skills that you must continue to nurture in all your professional life.

CONSEQUENCES OF USING POWER

One consequence of power is accountability. When an individual exercises power in relation to health care, that person is answerable for the results that were controlled. When results are positive, accountability enables a person to grow in self-esteem and be recognized for strengths and abilities. Others may provide positive feedback that enhances feelings of being valued. Thus, self-esteem is seen both as a resource for power and as a consequence of power used successfully. Power becomes self-sustaining in this respect.

Accountability is not always a welcome consequence. The person who is accountable must be prepared to accept the fact that mistakes and errors can be made. It is distressing to evaluate oneself as unsuccessful or less competent. Power in this instance would tend to diminish, because a resource for power, self-esteem, is diminished. If you accept accountability, you may need to be accountable for improving your own practice, for increasing your own ability, and for directing your own growth.

A change in personal relationships is also a possible consequence of power. Those who had previously been in a position of control may resent the loss of control or be threatened that control will be exerted over them. This is particularly true if one views power in terms of control over others rather than in terms of control over oneself and over outcomes. Thus, some relationships may be lost.

New personal relationships may be gained as a consequence of developing power. Those who see power as positive and valuable may wish a closer relationship with a powerful person. Individuals who agree with your goals and direction may align themselves with you.

POLITICAL POWER

We must be aware that decisions about health care funding and priorities increasingly are being made in the political rather than in the health care arena. To influence these decisions, nurses must be politically aware and active. The American Nurses' Association (ANA) and the National League for Nursing (NLN) have supported the development of political education through their publications and speakers. Representatives of the ANA and NLN testify before congressional committees on matters important to health care and to the practice of nursing. State and district nurses' associations perform the same functions at their levels. Individual nurses have used their expertise to testify before governmental bodies.

Nurses have also joined efforts in political action organizations that actively lobby and support candidates. The national political action group for nursing, called ANA-PAC, has been raising money for campaigns and in other ways assisting those congressional candidates who have professed views and beliefs supportive of health care goals.

SUMMARY

As we look back and summarize this information on power, we want to emphasize that power is a positive valuable asset for nurses. It can best be defined as the ability to accomplish desired ends. Power can be measured and those with more power are able to accomplish more. Both personal and material resources are important to the development of power. You need self-esteem, energy, enthusiasm, and a positive approach to life. Your abilities in problem solving and decision making are crucial to your attainment of power.

There are seven different types of power: legitimate, referent, reward, expert, coercive, connection, and information. You may increase your own power by using any of these types of power as well as by developing your own personal resources for power. Power is used through interpersonal interaction. You can best accomplish your desired goals by working with and through others. They are most likely to cooperate when you are willing to give to them and their efforts.

The use of power has many different consequences. Some of these, such as increased self-esteem, are positive; others, such as accountability for mistakes or errors, are more problematic. Personal relationships may also change when you achieve and exercise power.

Political power is also important for nurses. Nurses are becoming more and more aware of the need to be involved where basic funding and priority decisions are being made. Through working both individually and collectively, they are finding that they can affect the political process.

Study Questions/Activities

1.   Write your personal definition of power.
2.   List and define seven types of power.
3.   Identify a powerful person in your current work setting. Examine that person's background and list types of power used by that individual.
4.   List types of power that you currently possess and explain why you believe that you possess them.
5.   Devise a plan for increasing your personal power through increasing your resources for power and developing different types of power.
6.   Identify one goal you would like to see accomplished in your current work environment. Identify ways you could use your power to work toward attainment of that goal.
7.   Identify one possible adverse consequence of the use of power and identify ways in which you could overcome this adverse consequence.

REFERENCES

Bierstedt, R. (1950). An analysis of social power. *Advances in Nursing Science, 4*(5), 1–17.

Claus, K.E., & Bailey, J.T. (1977). *Power and influence in health care: A new approach to leadership.* St. Louis: C.V. Mosby.

Dahl, R. (1957). The concept of power. *Behavioral Science,* 2(3), 201–215.

French, J., & Raven, B. (1965). The bases of social power. In D. Cartwright & A. Lander (Eds.), *Studies in social power.* Ann Arbor: Institute for Social Research.

Hersey, P., Blanchard, K., & Natemeyer, W. (1979). *Situational leadership, perception, and the impact of power.* LaJolla, Calif.: Learning Resources Corporation.

Hesse–Biber, S. & Williamson, J. (1984). Resource theory and power in families: Life cycle considerations. *Family Processes,* 23(2), 261–278.

Josefowitz, N. (1980). *Paths to power: A woman's guide from first job to top executive.* Reading, Mass.: Addison-Wesley.

May, R. (1972) *Power and Influence.* New York: W.W. Norton and Co. Inc.

Molloy, J. (1988). *The new dress for success.* New York: Warner Books.

Petrellis, A.J. (1985). Using power in interactions with peers. *Supervisory Management,* 30(2), 19–25.

Random House Dictionary of the English Language. (1985). J. Stein (Ed.). New York: Random House.

Stevenson, J.S. (1982). Construction of a scale to measure load, power, and margin in life. *Nursing Research,* 31(4), 222–225.

Tannenbaum, A.S. & Cooke, R.A. (1974). Control and participation. *Journal of Contemporary Business,* 3, 35–46.

SUGGESTIONS FOR FURTHER READING

Barnum, B.J. (1988). Power: We love to talk about it. *Nursing and Health Care,* 10(10), 531.

Copp, L.A. (1989). That which empowers. *Journal of Professional Nursing,* 5(4), 169–170.

Del Bueno, D.J. (1987). How well do you use power? *American Journal of Nursing,* 87(11), 1495–1496.

Hoelzel, C.B. (1989). Using structural power sources to increase influence. *Journal of Nursing Administration,* 19(11), 10–15.

Lang, N.M. (1989). Empower the nurse: A time for renewal. *Nursing practice in the 21st century,* ANA Publ. CH-18, 5–16.

Maas, M.L. (1988). A model of organizational power: Analysis and significance to nursing. *Research in Nursing and Health,* 11(3), 153–163.

Smith, G.R. (1989). Speaking out: More power to you. *American Journal of Nursing,* 89(3), 357–358.

Strasen, L. (1989). Redesigning patient care to empower nurses and increase productivity. *Nursing Economics,* 7(1), 32–35.

Trofino, J. (1989) Empowering nurses. *Journal of Nursing Administration,* 19(4), 13.

Wiley, E.L. (1987) Acquiring and using power effectively. *Journal of Continuing Education,* 18(1), 25–28.

Facilitating the Management Process

II

Certain knowledge and skills, adequately understood and appropriately applied, may be viewed as facilitating the management process. Unit 2 discusses major topics that facilitate the management process. Learning to manage resources responsibly is critical for any new graduate. Developing skills in the decision-making process may make the difference in whether you receive a promotion or whether the position is given to someone else. Similarly, it is critical that you learn to manage your time wisely. The material presented in the chapter on time management will be as useful in your life outside the health care environment as it is within. Being able to motivate others to do their best job and to remain challenged by everyday responsibilities may make the difference between an effective manager and an ineffective one. Teaching staff is a day-to-day activity for any individual accountable for the care of a group of patients. Thus, you will find in this unit information that will facilitate your role as manager and coordinator of nursing care.

Managing Resources

5

Objectives

After completing this chapter, you should be able to:

1. *Describe the differences between operating and capital budgets.*
2. *Identify steps in the budget process.*
3. *Increase awareness of the costs associated with health care.*
4. *Determine the role of the nurse in cost containment.*
5. *Explain the relationship between cost awareness and cost containment.*
6. *Provide examples of cost containment measures related to the use of human and material resources.*

There was a time, prior to 1972, when most nurses in the health care system were oblivious to the costs associated with care, services, and supplies. Sterile gloves, sterile dressings, catheters, suction equipment, medications, and so on, were stocked on shelves and never charged to patients. Often stacks of sterile dressings were taken into patients' rooms and were later discarded if they were not needed. Although this behavior is considered wasteful now, it was common practice in the past.

The cost of health care has increased, and proportionally the money available for health care has decreased. There are many reasons for this rapid increase in cost. Increased regulation of health care facilities and providers has increased accountability for maintaining quality standards. Meeting these standards is costly but provides protection to the public. As the average age of our population has increased, so has the need for health care. These increases have required the system to stretch resources to meet demand. Use of new technology is often demanded by consumers of health care and quickly becomes the standard of practice for diagnosis and treatment. The cost of research for and development of this technology, purchase of equipment, and provision of knowledgeable personnel to operate it escalates the cost of care for everyone. Ethical questions arise related to distribution of scarce resources among an ever-increasing number of individuals.

The escalating cost of health care is the responsibility of all members of the health care team. Nurses do not have control of all elements that impact on health care costs, but they do have control over certain resources in the clinical setting; and to be cost effective they must use these resources responsibly. Nurses "should be aware of . . . what things cost, how they are paid for, how they are budgeted, how waste creeps in; how feelings affect results, and how money influences services. And, once aware, we should demand our say in planning; finances are too important to be left to the money men!" (Bluestone, 1973, p. 28).

Nurse managers, such as directors or vice presidents of nursing, supervisors, and head nurses, are often directly involved in communication with others in the organization regarding resource allocation. The bedside nurse is directly involved with and in control of utilization of resources for each patient. The nurse must maximize the resources available and recognize when resources are scarce and patient safety is jeopardized by their absence.

Although most often thought of in terms of money, resources also include supplies, personnel, and time. Cost effectiveness begins with cost awareness in all these areas.

WHERE DOES THE MONEY COME FROM?

The money for health care services comes primarily from three sources: the government, insurance companies, and "self pay," which means that the patient pays directly. The largest number of health care dollars is invested by the federal government. This includes Medicare reimbursement and grant funding for research and development of new products and methods for providing care. Those who do not have insurance and cannot afford to pay for health care may be eligible for Medicaid, which is a reimbursement system for the indigent funded by the federal and state governments. Federal funds also support the National Institutes for Health. Many Americans do have health insurance, which they select from a variety of options to cover their health care needs. Some can afford to "pay as they go" and prefer not to pay the premiums for an insurance policy. An increasing concern is the large number of individuals not covered by any insurance or governmental program who cannot afford health care.

In the 1950s, consumers began to purchase health insurance in large numbers (Strasen, 1987). These third-party payors intervened between the recipient of services and the bill, decreasing the patient's direct responsibility for payment. In the 1960s, workplace benefits usually included payment of health care insurance, which effectively distanced the consumer from the cost of care. The feeling that unlimited medical care should be available to all was perpetuated. Costs continued to escalate as high-technology advances became the standard of care.

The Medicare program was introduced under the Social Security Act of 1965 to provide health care insurance to individuals over the age of 65 and the disabled. Health care costs continued to escalate, although there were attempts to provide controls and decrease the government's bill for health care.

The consumer movement in the 1970s led to increased accountability and increased demand for all available medical services. Litigation during this time increased, and physicians and hospitals began to practice defensive medicine. Patients had tests they might not have needed in order to rule out esoteric diagnoses. The overall cost of health care increased further.

When voluntary efforts at cost control were not successful in the 1970s, the Tax Equity and Fiscal Responsibility Act was passed in October 1982. It changed the financial structure of health care institutions significantly. Limitations were placed on payments in a variety of areas, including outpatient services and nursing salary adjustments for working the evening and night shifts. Payments of hospital bills were made after services were rendered and were designed to reimburse for all expenses incurred (Simms, Price, & Ervin, 1985.)

The introduction of Diagnostic Related Groups (DRGs) in the Social Security Amendments of 1983 brought with it the concept of prospective reimbursement for Medicare and Medicaid recipients. Prospective reimbursement is a predetermined payment schedule, based on the average number of days of hospitalization for a specific diagnosis. It includes the expected costs for laboratory fees, various therapies, and surgery. If a patient stays more than the predetermined number of days, the hospital absorbs the cost or may request consideration for the additional expense. This was expected to balance with those staying less than the average number of days. In reality, hospitals believed that the payment schedule did not support care beyond the DRG-allocated days and began changing practices to encourage early discharge. Some private insurance companies also began instituting prospective reimbursement. In addition to the change in reimbursement, many procedures were designated as outpatient procedures, and inpatient care for performing them was denied. Prospective reimbursement has revolutionized the health care delivery system, resulting in fewer patient days of stay per diagnostic category and an increased need for home health care and outpatient diagnostic tests and surgery (Strasen, 1987). Hospitals responded to the threat of decreased income and decreased days of stay in many ways.

The increased acuity level of patients during their shortened stay created an increased demand for nurses in the hospital. The shift to outpatient procedures and convalescence in the home also increased the need for nurses outside of the hospital, thereby increasing the overall demand for nurses.

Reimbursement by third-party payors—including health insurance companies, health maintenance organizations, and federal and state government—and direct payment by patients make up the largest percentage of income to a hospital.

COST AWARENESS

Cost awareness is the first step in the process of cost containment. Expenditures in the budget of the nursing department are made up primarily of personnel costs and supply costs. The percentage of each of these in the budget varies with the inflationary spiral associated with the cost of supplies or the organizational climate permitting salary increases.

Most health care organizations are nonprofit, which means that all excess income over expenses is used within the organization to improve and/or expand services (Strasen, 1987). The viability, or survival and growth, of an organization can only be maintained by having more income than expenses.

Have you ever thought of yourself as an FTE? Nursing service administrators often refer to FTEs, by which they mean full-time equivalent employees in a position that can be equated to 40 hours per week times 52 weeks, for a total of 2080 hours per year (Hanson, 1983). An FTE is a unit of time and can be divided into parts. Half an FTE (0.5 FTE) is therefore equivalent to an employee working 20 hours per week. The important part of this equation is that one FTE is equivalent to 40 hours of employment per week whether worked by one full time person or several part time persons.

The total hours for an FTE include both productive and nonproductive time. Productive time is the time spent working on the unit; nonproductive time is that for which the employee is paid for not working, such as vacation time, sick leave, annual leave, and so forth. Nonproductive time varies, depending on the benefits of the employing institution. The nonproductive time subtracted from 2080 yields the productive work hours.

Calculation of "Nonproductive" Time

2 Weeks vacation	=	80 hr
12 Sick days	=	96 hr
10 Holidays	=	80 hr
2 Staff development days	=	16 hr

Total "nonproductive" time = 272 hr
2080 hr − 272 hr = 1808 hr for direct patient care

The 272 hours of nonproductive time must then be included in another position and must be considered in the budgeting process. Some labor costs are considered fixed; others may vary, depending upon the number and acuity of patients. Each hour counts and must be used wisely for cost containment. You can easily see that time is money and that those who arrive late, take extended lunch periods and coffee breaks, and are in the lounge when they should be working are squandering resources.

When labor costs are under control, the next area of concern is buying and distributing supplies. Economies of scale, otherwise known as volume buying, become important, as does appropriate conservation of supplies. It is a goal of the health care setting to provide safe, effective care at the lowest cost per patient day.

WHAT IS A BUDGET?

Basically, a budget is a formal plan presented in a document that indicates the expected income and expected expenses of the organization, department, or individual (Marriner-Tomey, 1988). Just as you balance your checkbook, the health care organization must balance its budget.

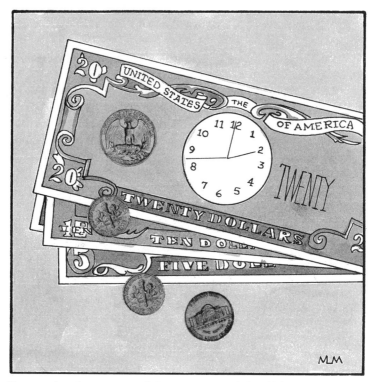

Because time is money, each hour counts and should be used wisely.

The budget allows the organization to plan and manage programs and control spending. Following the determination of the organization's goals and objectives by the Board of Trustees, the budget allows the organization to proceed with the master plan. The ability of the organization to meet its objectives within the budget parameters is a criterion often used to evaluate the overall performance of those responsible for the success and continued function of the organization. In addition to being a financial master plan, the budget is used to control and evaluate the organization's performance related to financial responsibility.

THE BUDGET PROCESS

The budget process and procedures vary from organization to organization. However, some parts of the process are common to all organizations. These include steps to gather information prior to budget preparation, such as environmental assessment, statement of mission and objectives, assumptions about the future, setting of operational objectives, preparation of budget manuals, and preparation of projection packages. Actual budget preparation then begins and includes completion of departmental budgets, departmental budget hearings, presentation of the institutional budget to the Finance Committee of the Board of Trustees, implementation of the operational budget, analysis of budget variances, year-end evaluation, and environmental assessment (Strasen, 1987). Does this remind you of the nursing process—assess, plan, implement, evaluate, and revise? The budget process is logical and something that we can easily follow.

Environmental assessment for budget purposes includes the environments that are both internal and external to the organization. The planners will identify the strengths and weakness of the organization, which might include such things as results of patient satisfaction surveys. The external environment takes into account the changing needs of the population in the area, including the shift in third-party payment patterns that might result in a change in focus of services offered. For example, the increase in the demand for outpatient procedures and home care has brought with it organizational responses that include increasing the number of outpatient surgical suites, enlarging waiting areas, providing adequate equipment and supplies, and increasing staffing. Acute-care organizations are planning to provide diverse services as they expand to include home health care, hospice care, adult day care, and others.

As a nurse, you can identify nursing needs in the community and develop a "product" to meet that need. Traditionally nurses have not thought of their services as a product. However, as the health care industry has become more competitive, the jargon used has taken on a marketing flair. The development of "product lines" has become commonplace.

The Board of Trustees establishes the direction for the institution through the mission and goal statements. An example of a goal statement is, "To provide health care services that respond to the changing demographics of the community served." A statement such as this will provide direction for future planning and expansion of services. Assumptions and projections about the future are incorporated in environmental planning and statements of objectives. (See Chapter 1 for more discussion of mission and goals.)

The operational objectives are the more specific objectives of each department and are reflected in the unit goals. The nursing department is involved in interpreting the implications of increasing the number of outpatient surgical suites or providing home health care services as they relate to the nursing budget. Nurse managers in various areas generally seek input from those working for them. If you are concerned with making suggestions for improvement or change, developing an objective appropriate to the unit and consistent with organizational objectives is a good way to begin (see Chap. 3).

Because all those involved in the budget process must "speak the same language," a budget manual is usually provided by the chief financial officer to provide definitions of terms and appropriate forms and examples. This provides for consistent format and comparison of documents among departments. The language of a budget manual is often difficult to decipher. You will not be expected to understand the entire process, but it will be helpful to be aware of various parts of the budget and the percentage of money distributed in each category.

To estimate the available funds for the upcoming fiscal year, projections based on prior history of patient days, and assumptions about such things as future growth or shifts in services are prepared. Generally, the Director of Nursing will work with the financial officer to develop projections specific to the department.

Department budgets are done yearly for the following fiscal year. Salaries and benefits, supplies and equipment are the major areas of concern. Departmental hearings are held within the department to help in further establishing priorities within the unit and assuring that they are reflected as priorities in the budget document. Nurses on the unit may provide input to this process, either directly or indirectly, depending upon the system established at the institution. Hearings often include a review of the budget of the prior year, achievement of goals, and the relationship of one budget year to the next.

Once all the departments present and justify their budgets to the financial and executive officers of the institution, the budget is presented to the Finance Committee, which reviews the document to determine if it meets the institutional goals. At this time additional changes or review may be requested. The budget is generally brought to the committee several months prior to the expected date of implementation, so that adequate time is provided for changes. If revisions are made, the Finance Committee will review the document again. Following acceptance from the Finance Committee, the document is presented for final approval to the Board of Trustees, which then authorizes expenditure of funds as presented for the next fiscal year.

The work of the members of the Finance Committee is not complete at this point, however, because it is their function to monitor the budget at least monthly; identify variances between the projected and actual revenue and expenses; and request explanations, changes, or additional information as needed. The terminology at this point can be confusing. *Variance* is simply the difference between the projected budget for expenses and the actual expenses incurred. A variance of increased revenue over expenses is a positive variance. Lower expenditure than expected in relation to the budgeted expenses is also viewed as a positive variance. In terms of nursing, a nursing shortage results in fewer hours being paid for; therefore, actual expenses are significantly less than budgeted expenses.

This also is referred to as a positive variance, although the impact is actually quite negative.

The Finance Committee reviews the budget each month, but at the completion of the fiscal year there is additional overview. The progress of the organization in using the established tools and meeting the objectives in a cost-effective manner is evaluated, and the assumptions about the future are reviewed. The process then begins again! The budget process is constant and ongoing.

OPERATING AND CAPITAL BUDGETS

The total organizational budget is usually separated into two distinct sections: the *operating budget* and the *capital budget*. "The operating budget is concerned with expendable items or those with a short usable life" (Rowland & Rowland, 1980, p. 180)—those that are used in the day-to-day operation of the institution, such as supplies and salaries. Supplies include such things as books and magazines, sterile packs for various procedures, gloves, syringes, linen, pens, and pencils. Unexpected items often included under supplies include copying and equipment rental.

Items to be included in the capital budget are usually listed in the budget manual. The capital budget expenditures include major equipment or changes in the physical plant requiring modification, renovation, or construction. The budget manual for an organization will stipulate an arbitrary amount, such as $300, that defines a capital expenditure. Supplies that cost more than $300 per item would then be included in the capital budget. Remodeling costs above $300 may also be capital expenditures. If, for example, doorways needed to be widened to allow wheelchair access, the renovation costs may be reflected in the capital budget.

The budget for supplies is usually calculated by using the prior year as a baseline, determining a projected expansion or decrease in associated services, and adding a predetermined expected rate of inflation. The budget for supplies can be significantly affected by increasing attention to conservation, decreasing the supplies needed, or decreasing the cost per unit. Smaller hospitals often combine efforts to increase volume purchasing and decrease the cost of each item.

WHAT IS THE NURSE'S ROLE?

The Joint Commission for the Accreditation of Health Care Organizations developed the following guidelines, which have served to encourage nurses' input into the budget process (Fuller, 1976):

1. The objectives of nursing care are utilized as determinants in forecasting the nursing service budget.
2. Nursing personnel directly involved in practice provide estimates of projected budgetary needs.
3. Nursing administration reviews and analyzes reports of its financial operation on an ongoing basis and shares information with nursing staff.
4. The budget is evaluated and revised as necessary by the nursing administration on the basis of available resources and program priorities.

Nurse participation in the budget process is thereby mandated.

Cost awareness, in terms of time, materials, and money, begins at the bedside. The nurse carefully balances the quality of care with conservative management of available resources. It is the legal responsibility of the nurse to maintain the standard of care and not jeopardize patient safety. This "balancing act" takes planning. It is just as important for the staff nurse to plan carefully how his or her time will be divided among six assigned patients as it is for the head nurse to plan for the unit.

Time is a valuable resource. It is important to be concerned with the way you organize your own time as well as the way you delegate to others assisting with nursing care. As salaries of nurses increase, hospital man-

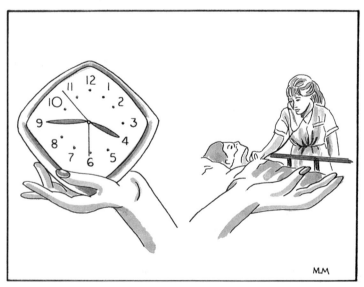

It is just as important for the staff nurse to plan carefully how time will be divided among assigned patients as it is for the head nurse to plan for the unit.

agement will become more concerned with the tasks usually assigned to nurses that might be done by lower-paid personnel. The art of delegation of appropriate nursing tasks must be mastered (see Chap. 7). Appropriate supervision of those to whom you delegated is essential. Developing a team approach and commitment to quality care will help in getting all members of the team to recognize the importance of using time efficiently. Keep in mind that employees who do not give a full day's work for a full day's pay cost the institution (and eventually the patient) additional money. The arts of supervision and motivation become very important elements in deescalating the cost of health care.

You should realize that meetings are expensive and must be planned carefully. Remember that a 1-hour meeting with eight people amounts to 8 man-hours, or 1 working day, so it is essential to plan the meeting and make it worthwhile. A 1-hour meeting of eight nurses who earn an average salary of $20 per hour costs at least $160. If additional staff members are needed while the nurses are in the meeting, the cost of that additional staff must also be factored in.

Nurses can also determine if a routine is outmoded or no longer needed. Repetitious paperwork might be reduced, especially with the introduction of computers. You, as a staff nurse, can make recommendations to streamline the system at the grassroots level. You are the best one to evaluate existing systems and anticipate needed changes.

Cost containment measures apply to the use of material and human resources. Material resources include supplies and equipment. The nursing and purchasing departments must communicate well to determine the best product for the intended use. The lowest bidder may provide a product that breaks easily, is difficult to open, is undependable, and needs to be repaired frequently. If those who work with the equipment do not inform them, people in the purchasing department will remain unaware of these problems. In fact, the lowest bid may in the long run be more expensive in terms of wasted time and frustration. Providing clear product specifications for those who purchase the products is the first step in a cooperative effort toward cost effectiveness.

EXAMPLE: NURSING SERVICE OPERATING BUDGET— COMMUNITY HOSPITAL

The budget year for many organizations ends on June 30. The planning process for the budget begins many months before. At Community Hospital the planning process for the next fiscal year (beginning July 1) begins in January, when the finance office prepares the budget packets for distribution to department managers. The budget packets are distributed during February and returned to the finance office by the end of March. During February and March the area managers become familiar with the worksheets and policies and procedures provided in the packet and begin to coordinate budget needs within their areas. During April the departmental budget requests are compiled, summarized, and presented to the Budget Committee for review. The Budget Committee then meets with the department managers to discuss the budget requests. The discussions focus on both the operational and financial issues relevant to each department. Projected revenues are balanced against projected expenses. Once approved, the budget is forwarded to the Board of Trustees for final approval and oversight.

Once you are familiar with important dates in the budget review for the organization with which you are involved, you can provide timely input. There are few things more frustrating than being told that additional personnel or supplies cannot be obtained, because they were not budgeted!

At Community Hospital, the best time to provide input from the grassroots level is in February and March, when the department manager is working on the budget. Providing rationale and backup information regarding your recommendation will be helpful, because the manager can then be well prepared, with your help, to defend the budget change or increase.

It is helpful to be aware of the definitions included in the budget package. There is often a fine line between supplies and equipment. In some institutions the differentiation is made based on cost; for example, supplies that cost more than $300 may be categorized as equipment. Because supplies are included in the operating budget and equipment is included in the capital budget and the budget justification schedules may differ, it is important to know the category into which your request falls.

Budgets are less intimidating when you are familiar with the format and the process. Table 5–1 is a typical Nursing Service Operating Budget Summary. The actual department budget provides, in greater detail, the items that make up the final total in each category. The budget summary is a composite of the budgets submitted by each nursing unit.

Table 5–2 shows a sample worksheet used for medical/surgical supplies for a nursing unit.

The best time for a staff nurse to have input into the budget is during the preparation of the worksheet. The example includes only some of the supplies that are needed on a daily basis. If a need for additional supplies is projected, then this is the time to include it.

A staff nurse can become directly involved in the budget process through participation on unit, area, or departmental budget committees and/or through providing legitimate and timely budget requests.

TABLE 5–1. SUMMARY OF OPERATING EXPENSES FOR NURSING SERVICES (BUDGET YEAR ENDING JUNE 30, 1990)

Cost Center Description	FTEs	Salaries	Med/Surg Supplies	Non Med/Surg Supplies	Purchased Services	Professional Fees	Other Direct Expenses	Total
Unit 3	21.20	$541,519	$19,551	$23,657	$660	$0	$5,730	$591,117
Unit 1	16.36	513,668	24,960	4,569	910	0	925	545,032
Alcohol rehab	24.50	670,596	2,100	22,420	24,620	0	21,913	741,649
Unit 4	30.73	960,714	42,062	9,803	0	0	275	1,012,854
Unit 5	41.70	1,204,035	59,664	7,830	180,350	0	720	1,452,599
Unit 2	32.24	1,063,195	54,367	12,212	0	0	400	1,130,174
Unit 3	30.04	983,326	54,151	9,437	0	0	270	1,047,184
Unit 5	38.40	1,185,577	51,355	8,677	100	0	650	1,246,359
Float pool—education	0.00	86,946	0	0	0	0	0	86,946
Alcohol detox	25.50	597,698	6,323	6,476	0	0	200	610,697
Sleep center	2.00	50,101	395	103	8,140	0	0	58,739
Cardiology center	43.82	1,540,217	75,445	10,029	2,438	0	2,642	1,630,771
Cancer center	1.00	38,486	0	1,479	1,008	25,000	2,500	68,473
Critical care unit	46.45	1,684,214	92,816	10,437	1,000	0	1,572	1,790,039
Psychiatry	29.80	886,457	7,456	17,487	3,563	40,000	4,733	959,696
Operating room	56.79	1,702,956	2,121,620	150,146	62,056	0	600	4,037,378
Post anesthesia care unit	19.90	723,711	22,274	5,547	0	0	405	751,937
Ambulatory surgery	22.74	632,982	219,196	45,423	27,630	0	600	925,831
Medical endoscopy	3.50	118,766	15,175	11,999	16,980	0	300	163,220
SHA urgent care	5.20	211,097	8,355	3,559	37,660	25,200	44,270	330,141
ER—medical	31.09	1,125,262	158,167	50,178	8,430	2,800	19,648	1,364,485
Cardiac rehab	3.16	93,927	2,315	6,419	6,630	1,500	7,367	118,158
Anesthesiology	0.00	0	350,600	6,275	21,857	0	0	378,732
Nursing adminstration	19.93	596,624	108	16,855	10,981	500	7,842	632,910
Clinical specialists	7.00	254,933	190	2,352	305	0	2,564	260,344
Diabetic pt. instruction	1.77	61,941	988	4,277	4,290	0	5,176	76,672
IV therapy	9.00	318,444	26,147	754	0	0	400	345,745
Nursing services	561.82	$17,847,393	$3,415,780	$448,400	$419,608	$95,000	$131,702	$22,357,882

TABLE 5–2. MEDICAL/SURGICAL SUPPLIES (BUDGET YEAR 19___–19___)

SCHEDULE
4–1

Pg. _2_ of _6_
Department Number _6340_   Department Name _CCLL_

Expense Code	Vendor	Description	Quantity	Cost per Item	Total Cost	Expense Code Total
452	Storeroom	PRN Adaptors	2600	.63	1638	
	''	Teflon Guidewires	50	9.26	463	
	''	Cordis Introducers	50	14.25	712	6003
467	Pharmacy	Heparin Flush Kits–210/Boxes	—	68.68	15726	
		Stock Drugs Insulin, ASA, Tylenol		575.00	575	16,321
490	Storeroom	Chemstrips	70/Boxes	23.55	1648	
	''	Cultureittes	150	.54	81	
	''	Gowns & Mask	700	1.73	1211	
	''	Adult Diapers	200	.35	70	
	''	Posey & Mitts	200	2.02	404	
	''	Urine Clean Catch	225	.70	157	
	''	Hemosult Kits	8	42.66	341	

THE ROLE OF THE NURSE IN COST CONTAINMENT

An ethical question arises with regard to the quality of care that limited funding can support. When analyzing this precarious balance, the quality, efficiency, effectiveness, and cost must be factored into the decision. The effectiveness and efficiency of the use of resources, other than money, must also be monitored as carefully as the total budget. If successful, these efforts will result in lowered costs and increased patient satisfaction (Ehrat, 1987). Efforts may be made on an agency-wide basis by the administration, on a unit-wide basis, and by the individual nurse. Of course, to be most effective, all levels should be participating.

Traditionally, the cost of nursing care has been included on the patient's bill as an integral part of "room and board," as are housekeeping, maintenance, and other services. It is becoming increasingly important to determine the actual costs of nursing care, independent from other costs. Although controversy exists regarding whether nursing services should be billed separately, it is agreed that separating out cost of nursing services is essential to increase accountability for efficient and cost-effective care. It is also agreed that when resources are scarce, there is increased competition for them. To be more competitive in this environment, it becomes important to demonstrate the ability to generate income. In economic terms, the nursing department becomes a profit center, rather than a cost center that indicates only the dollars expended (Ullman & Plevak, 1988).

Exacting tools have not yet been developed that specifically identify nursing costs. Most frequently, an institution determines total nursing costs and direct nursing costs. Direct nursing costs reflect the intensity of nursing care that can be measured in time required and supplies used; they include assessment, planning, implementation, and evaluation of nursing care (Ullman & Plevak, 1988). Total nursing costs include the cost of support personnel and services, including staff development, supervisors, liaison nurses, and specialty nurses, such as enterostomal therapists.

Some organizations are now working on developing systems for charging for nursing care. Most of these projects use patient classification systems as a basis for determining the level of nursing care required and therefore the hours of nursing care needed. It then becomes possible to determine the cost of care by multiplying the number of nursing hours anticipated by the average nursing salary.

Patient classification systems can also be used to determine appropriate staffing levels. The average number of nursing hours required per month could then be used to project the number of hours of nursing care and therefore the number of FTEs needed. If the acuity level increases overall, requiring additional hours of care, a float pool of nursing staff or

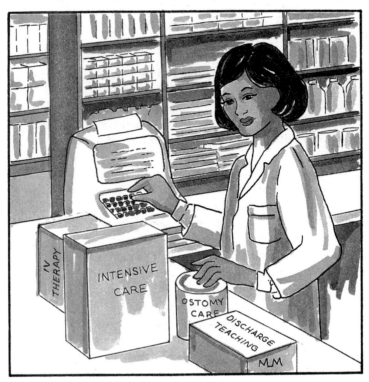

Determining the actual cost of nursing care independent from other costs becomes increasingly important.

temporary nurse pools can be used to supplement the projected need. The effectiveness of this type of system, although generally initiated by administration, depends upon the direct input of the nurse who provides patient care and who determines the patient's acuity level at least one time per day.

Determination of the use of cost accounting and patient classification systems is generally made at the administrative level. Another administrative decision is whether nurses should share directly in the decision making. Shared governance is an organizational approach that allows staff nurses to share in administrative decisions. A staff nurse can share ideas directly while serving on committees dealing with quality of care, personnel issues, scheduling, recruitment, and even budget and finance. If you are interested in being involved with direct decision making, when you are looking for a job you should ask about the governance process.

Independent of the larger organization, the nurse manager of a unit, with staff input, can develop efficient systems for an individual unit.

Successful innovations that began on one "experimental" unit can then be used on other units. Documentation provides a good example, because it is often an area that gets a good deal of attention and is time-consuming. From the legal perspective, nurses are told that courts of law assume that if something is not charted, it was not done. But when the process of documentation is analyzed, it is often found that descriptive charting causes duplication of information (Murphy & Beglinger, 1988). Is it necessary to indicate in a narrative note that vital signs are normal when, in fact, a graphic or flow sheet already includes that information? It has also been found that unnecessary transcription of information from one sheet to another, as often occurs with vital signs, contributes greatly to overtime and therefore to increasing the cost of care (Murphy & Beglinger, 1988).

To tackle this problem, a unit might implement guidelines for narrative charting by exception and then design flow sheets that provide documentation of routine and normal findings and procedures and nursing care most frequently performed on that unit. Charting by exception is the narrative documentation of abnormal or significant findings. Murphy and Begliner found that with traditional charting methods, RNs average 44 minutes per shift, versus 25 minutes per shift with charting by exception. This may not sound like much, but if there are 350 nurses, and each saves 19 minutes, then the total gain in time is more than 110 hours per day (Murphy & Beglinger, 1988)!

The employing institution, and even the nursing unit, might adopt cost-containing policies and procedures, but in the end the individual nurse must implement them. Commitment to cost containment is supported by the philosophy that if everyone does his part, the cumulative effect will be great. It is therefore important for you to do your part, no matter how insignificant it seems.

One of the first things a nurse can do is to choose a job carefully. It is also important for the employing agency to place new graduates carefully to maximize potential and encourage job satisfaction. The orientation cost for new staff is high. Maintaining staff and increasing retention of employees decreases the need for orientation sessions. By choosing carefully, you are more likely to become committed to the organization. As you remain in the position and feel comfortable, you begin to develop short-term and long-term professional goals.

Many experts feel that the direct care givers can make the greatest impact on quality of care and cost containment. One example cited by Barbara O'Brien in *Nursing Management* (1988) related to frustration of staff in the OR because OR table parts were frequently missing. Members of the staff worked together to solve the problem. Because it was estimated that it took 10 minutes per case to find the missing parts, not only was the staff more satisfied in solving the problem, but the total time saved allowed an additional case to be scheduled.

Legal and ethical standards for nursing care require adherence to standards of care defined by the profession. Standards of care and patient safety must not be compromised in the name of cost containment. A nurse who is aware of influences on the costs of health care can readily demonstrate to the organization that the use of old or contaminated supplies that cause the patient additional complications and result in an increase in the number of days of hospitalization is dollar foolish. The role of the nurse in "anticipatory management," which is reflected in the ability to assess a patient astutely and recognize problems before they become major, is critical to cost efficiency.

Several large hospitals have reported more than $1 million in losses from supplies that were used but not charged (Norton et al., 1988). The cost of these supplies was not recoverable from insurance reimbursement. Often documentation of procedures that were performed was inadequate and could not be used to justify the use of supplies. As a nurse you need to be familiar with the method of charging supplies, whether by bar-code directly into a computer, a charge slip, or stickers on a cardex (but not on your uniform pocket), and you must follow through with the process. You must also accurately document procedures and equipment used. A study in a large hospital found that supplies such as K-pads, wall suction, suction catheters, and underpads were among those frequently not charged (Norton et al., 1988.)

At this point you might wonder why it is so important to charge the patient for supplies, because the large hospital should be able to absorb the costs. In actuality, a not-for-profit hospital that must maintain and update equipment and services cannot afford to absorb costs. As a result, the cost of care for each patient is increased (Norton et al., 1988).

The nurse's ability to adjust to new policies related to charting practices, providing reports in ways that save time yet are more meaningful, such as "walking rounds," and adapting to new technology, all play an important part in cost containment. Awareness is the first step in decreasing work hours and increasing efficiency.

The development of management and communication skills, which allow the nurse to motivate others successfully to use their time and effort efficiently and become more aware of costs, has become a necessity.

SUMMARY

As the costs of health care increase because of such factors as inflation, increased use of technology, and increased demand on services by an aging population, it becomes more and more important to contain costs wherever possible. An individual nurse, whether at the bedside managing patient care, as a unit manager directing personnel, or in senior management setting policy, can have a great impact on the economics of health care. Awareness of costs associated with personnel, supplies, and equipment is the first step in cost containment. As a patient advocate the nurse is legally and ethically responsible for providing safe, competent care efficiently and effectively. If patient safety is compromised because of cost efficiency, the care provided is below standard and is not cost effective.

Medical costs are generally reimbursed by insurance companies, the government (in the form of Medicare or Medicaid), or the individual who pays the bill directly. In the 1980s the change in payment for services for patients covered under Medicare from a program that paid all charges following hospitalization to one that prepays the facility based on expected days of stay for a particular diagnostic category (DRG) changed the system drastically. Nurse managers became concerned with providing the best care in the shortest time at the lowest cost.

Nurses can become more aware of costs and where they can be decreased by an understanding of and direct involvement in the budget process. This also allows the nurse to influence allocations in the budget. The operating budget includes supplies and personnel essential for the day-to-day functioning of a unit. The capital budget includes certain supplies, equipment, and costs for changes in the physical plant. Each budget is reviewed separately. The Joint Commission on Accreditation of Health Care Organizations expects nurses to be involved in the budget process.

Nurses who are aware of costs are more likely to take cost-containing measures. Being aware of the use of time, supplies, and equipment will help to decrease the abuse of these resources. Time management skills, communication skills, and the ability to delegate tasks appropriately all play a part in cost containment. An individual nurse will be involved in cost containment on a daily basis. Providing input for the patient classification system, appropriately charging each item used for a patient, and developing efficient documentation methods are just a few of the things that can be done to contain costs.

A growing number of nurse executives feel that nurses could have a greater impact on the health care organization if nursing services were billed separately and the nursing department was viewed as producing income. This is an issue currently under investigation.

The savings generated by each nurse, though they may seem insignificant at the time, when multiplied by the number of nurses and the number of days in the year are substantial. The challenge is to find cost-effective, time-efficient methods of providing the best possible patient care.

Study Questions/Activities

1. For the health care organization with which you are most familiar, identify
   a. the fiscal year dates.
   b. critical dates in the budget cycle.
   c. the definition of supplies and equipment from the budget manual.
2. Using the information obtained for the preceding question, plan an appropriate strategy to have an IV monitor that costs $500 included in the budget. Consider
   a. justification for the purchase.
   b. whether this would be considered an operating or capital expense.
   c. an appropriate time line.
3. What is the cost of the following items needed for changing a sterile dressing:

	Cost to the hospital	Cost to the patient	Cost in the drugstore
a. Two sterile 4 × 4 pads	_____	_____	_____
b. One sterile combine pad	_____	_____	_____
c. 18″ of ¾″ hypoallergenic tape	_____	_____	_____
d. Three Betadine wipes	_____	_____	_____

4. For a hospital with which you are familiar, describe the opportunities available for nurses to participate in the budget process.

REFERENCES

Bluestone, N. (1973). One course Sue Barton never took: Health care economics. *American Journal of Nursing, 3*(11), 28.

Ehrat, K.S. (1987). The cost-quality balance: An analysis of quality, efficiency, and cost. *Journal of Nursing Administration, 17*(5), 12.

Fuller, M.E. (1976). The budget. *Journal of Nursing Administration, 6*(4), 36.

Hanson, R.L. (1983). *Management systems for nursing service staffing*. Rockville, Md.: Aspen Systems.

Marriner-Tomey, A. (1988). *Guide to nursing management,* 3rd ed. St. Louis: C.V. Mosby.

Murphy, J., & Beglinger, J.E. (1988). Charting by exception: Meeting the challenge of cost containment. *Nursing Management, 19*(2), 64.

Norton, V.M., Thorne, K., Bickerstaff, C., Kilgo, L., Pate, P., Cox, C., & Lawrence, D. (1988). Cost busters fair: Increasing staff awareness of cost effective practice. *Journal of Nursing Administration, 18*(9), 16–20.

O'Brien, B. (1988). QA: A commitment to excellence. *Nursing Management, 19*(11), 38.

Rowland, H.S., & Rowland, B.L. (1980). *Nursing administration handbook.* Rockville, Md.: Aspen Systems.

Simms, L., Price, S., & Ervin, N. (1985). *The professional practice of nursing administration.* New York: John Wiley.

Strasen, L. (1987). *Key business skills for nurse managers.* Philadelphia: J.B. Lippincott.

Ullman, S.G., & Plevak, M.L. (1988). Nursing units and profit centers: Survey and analysis. *Nursing Management, 19*(2), 64.

SUGGESTIONS FOR FURTHER READING

Donovan, M.I. et al. (1987). Costs of nursing services: Are the assumptions valid? *Nursing Administration 12*(1), 1–6.0.

McCarthy, C.M. (1988). DRGs—Five years later. *The New England Journal of Medicine, 318*(25), 1683–1686.

McClosky, J.C. (1989). Implications of costing out nursing services for reimbursement. *Nursing Management, 20*(1), 44–46, 48–49.

Reinhardt, U.E. (1988). In search of the magic bullet for climbing costs. *Hospitals, 62*(15), 22.

Skydell, B. et al. (1988). The price of nursing care. *Nursing Clinics of North America. 23*(3), 493–501.

Welch, H.G. & Larson, E.B. (1988). Dealing with limited resources: The Oregon decision to curtail funding for organ transplantation. *The New England Journal of Medicine, 319*(3), 171–173.

Decision Making for Patient Care

6

Objectives

After completing this chapter, you should be able to:

1. *Identify the reasons it is important for nurses to become effective decision makers.*
2. *List three advantages to a systematic and comprehensive decision-making process.*
3. *Identify the seven steps in the decision-making process.*
4. *Define terms relevant to the decision-making process, such as* responsibility, authority, feasible, *and* realistic.
5. *Describe how listing pros and cons can assist with decision making.*
6. *Discuss decision trees and decision grids.*
7. *Outline how numerical scoring can be used for decision making.*
8. *Discuss various participative approaches to decision making, including the task force, quality circles, brainstorming, the nominal group technique, and the Delphi method.*
9. *Identify characteristics of an effective decision maker.*
10. *Discuss guidelines for consistently making effective decisions.*

Decision making is a central component of the more general problem-solving process (assessment, problem statement, planning, implementation, and evaluation), which you studied as the nursing process. It is a cognitive process in which you must choose among alternatives. Often the best alternative of several courses of action is not clear. The decision-making process recommended in this chapter will help eliminate some uncertainty and make you more comfortable as you try to make effective decisions.

Effective decision making occurs when the process is conducted systematically and comprehensively and when the consequences of the implemented decision are determined (Barry, 1989). The most effective decision results in positive outcomes and fewer negative consequences. Goal-oriented analysis of the situation, its problems, and their alternative solutions are hallmarks of effective decision making (Duespohl, 1983).

A comprehensive and systematic approach to decision making has many advantages (Bailey & Claus, 1975). First, nurses will understand where they are in the process. Because it is systematic it will possess order, direction, guidance, and ongoing feedback. Second, a systematic approach provides a framework for gathering data relevant to the decision.

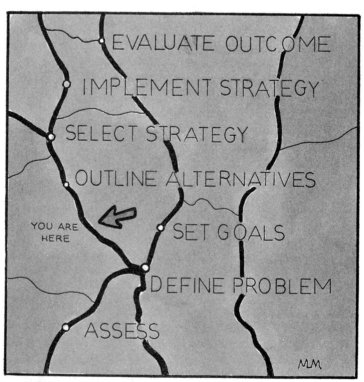

A comprehensive and systematic approach to decision making helps nurses understand where they are in the process.

Nurses will not waste time collecting irrelevant information. Third, nurses will be able to reach effective decisions based upon their previous knowledge, which will minimize errors and improve patient care.

THE CHALLENGE TO NURSES

Nurses have always been expected to make correct decisions. However, as recently as the 1960s, they were given limited information, authority, and reward for making them (Matteson & McConnell, 1988). In today's modern health care arena, especially in many institutional settings, nurses often have significant information, suitable authority, and ever-increasing compensation for the responsibility associated with decision making. Nurses are now required to consistently make effective decisions. This demand constitutes a challenge.

All nurses have managerial responsibilities of one type or another and therefore must make effective decisions that affect others as well as themselves. Their decisions cover a host of concerns—time management, resource allocation, interactions within the health care team, direct patient care, and many more—related to effectively managing the overall patient care environment.

Modern health care is concerned with the results a decision brings as well as with the costs of that decision (Roemer, 1986). Effective decisions are viewed as those that most quickly, simply, inexpensively, and fully achieve the desired outcome. Effective decisions help to contain overall costs and enhance productivity by facilitating the efficient use of both human and material resources. Unless nurses can meet this challenge by consistently making effective decisions, minimally productive activity will result.

You can see that effective decision making is an important skill for the nurse manager. Although some nurses appear to be born decision makers, most must learn and develop this skill. Nursing education, practice, management, and research have all recognized its importance and have promoted skilled decision making.

STEPS IN THE DECISION-MAKING PROCESS

There are many approaches to skillful decision making. Some authorities reduce it to as few as four steps (it is more commonly referred to as problem solving at this point); others identify 10 steps, all of which they think are necessary. Most of the models have similar steps, combined in some and separated in others. For our purposes we shall discuss a seven-step process. Taken cumulatively, these seven steps represent the decision-making process. However, it is important to realize that each step requires that one or more decisions be made for the process to proceed. This further implies that the steps must be taken in a particular sequence so that no details are overlooked.

Step 1: Assess the Situation

Before you can make a decision about a situation in a patient care environment, you must possess a complete and accurate understanding of that situation. To gain this information, the three following questions are frequently asked by nurses.

WHAT INFORMATION MUST I OBTAIN?   Usually this information concerns various needs in the patient care environment—those of the patient, the nurse, and other members of the health care team.

It also will include information concerning the institution and its resources. For each of these needs or types of needs, you must determine the degree to which the needs are satisfied, both how much and how well (Alfaro, 1986).

HOW DO I OBTAIN THIS INFORMATION?   In answering this question you will use methods for holistic assessment basic to nursing, including observation of the overall environment as well as observation and examination of the patient. This will include using good communication skills. The information will be obtained initially and will then be updated on an ongoing basis.

It is difficult to determine when you have enough information. You can never have all the information possible, but at some point you must determine you have enough and proceed to the next step in the decision-making process. You will also wonder if you have the right information. You may not learn the answer to this question until you reach the end of the decision-making process.

Frequently, when a nurse makes an ineffective decision, the fault lies with incomplete or inaccurate data obtained during this initial assessment. One should never minimize the importance of this initial assessment in the overall decision-making process.

WHAT DO I DO WITH THIS INFORMATION?   Once the data are collected, they must be processed. To make this information meaningful you must analyze and interpret it. Analysis and interpretation are fairly complicated human cognitive processes and are not easily understood. Prescott, Dennis, and Jacox (1987) suggest that you first analyze the individual pieces of the information as each piece relates to another and to your own knowledge base. They then recommend interpretation of the data through the process of association between pieces of data via human reasoning. Several additional suggestions can be made to facilitate effective analysis and interpretation of data.

First, think out loud, especially with a more experienced nurse or health care team member. They have had experience with the decision-making process and understand it.

Next, have the necessary information at your fingertips. This requires knowing your situation rather than guessing at pieces of information or fumbling through your notes.

Communicate your analysis and interpretation of the information to others who can be constructively critical; invite their comments. Encourage them to play the devil's advocate role.

Take your time (when you can). Fortunately, although data collection may be time-consuming, sometimes you may be able to understand the data more rapidly.

The result of these activities will be a holistic and informed view of the particular situation requiring a decision. You will know what you have and will be prepared to compare it with the desired situation.

Step 2: Define the Problem(s)

In step 2 you identify the actual or potential problems. In nursing process we refer to this step as the *diagnostic stage*. It requires the nurse to analyze and interpret, and it demands an ongoing, focused assessment of the situation, which you remember from the previous step. Aspinall and Tanner (1981, p. 5) state, "The problem identification phase is probably the most complex . . . and critical component [of the decision-making process] . . . the rest of the process will be successful only to the extent that the data base (and problems) are accurate and complete."

After the initial assessment, you have knowledge of the degree of fulfillment of the needs of those in the patient care environment. Problems are determined based on the degree to which these needs are met or fulfilled (Lewis, 1970). The *actual* problem represents a discrepancy between how well the need is currently being met and the ideal or desired fulfillment of that need. It might be represented by a deficiency in need fulfillment or an excess of need fulfillment. Although both types occur, deficiencies are the most common type (Johnson & Davis, 1975).

Working from this definition, we would define a *potential* problem as a danger that a discrepancy between the actual fulfillment of the need and the desired fulfillment of the need will occur at some time in the near future. To determine that a potential problem exists you must identify specific indicators that represent a danger.

How do we determine that problems actually exist? We must compare our assessment of this situation with what we know theoretically about the optimal situation. For example, if you have assessed the patient's blood pressure at 225/105 and you know from what you have learned in your nursing studies that 140/90 is generally considered a maximum reading, it is not difficult to identify a problem. Unfortunately, in many institutional situations a discrepancy will not be this clear. Furthermore, an analysis may yield multiple discrepancies.

We must now interpret the discrepancy or discrepancies and identify the actual or potential problems. Several guiding questions that will assist the nurse in this interpretation are listed in the accompanying display.

Now that you have a better picture of the need and the discrepancy, you must gather more information about it via a focused assessment. The assessment will be focused directly on the need(s) and will be more subjective, because you have a particular problem about which you are trying to learn more. The nurse's knowledge base is critical to the focused assessment, for the nurse must know what to assess. At this point we begin to examine rationale relevant to the problem. The focused assessment will assist you in clearly stating the problem in terms that are understandable to others.

Step 3: Determine Short-Term and Long-Term Goals

For each problem that has been identified, both long-term and short-term goals must be made and prioritized (Barry, 1989). This is not as simple as it sounds, because problems and goals overlap or occur in clusters that inhibit their prioritization. All problems may be important, but some are more important than others. Likewise, all goals are desired, but some are not as essential as others.

Guiding Questions in the Interpretation of Discrepancies

- *What* is the discrepancy?
- *Where* does it occur?
- *When* does it occur—how often and under what conditions or circumstances?
- *How* big is it?
- *Why* is this disicrepancy occurring?
- *What* am I going to do about it?

(Kepner, C., & Tregoe, B. [1985]. *The rational manager.* New York: McGraw-Hill.)

All problems (and the related goals) should be considered when establishing priorities, because what you see as the problem now may not be the problem later. Situations and patient care environments are dynamic; they change. The nurse's decision making must be responsive to this. You must conduct an ongoing assessment of the situation pertinent to each problem and set of goals you identify.

When setting down priorities, the nurse must consider the constraints, capabilities, and resources of the institution and environment (Bailey & Claus, 1975). The following are some of the factors the nurse should consider:

- The hierarchy of needs, problems, goals, and objectives
- The characteristics of all persons involved in the situation, including their overall bio-psycho-social needs and their motivation
- Factors within the environment itself, including the time available, the financial resources, the equipment and facilities, the personnel, and the philosophy of care.

Once the goals and priorities are developed, you are ready to proceed with the decision-making process. You will want to decide what you will need to do to meet the most critical goal.

Step 4: Analyze Alternative Strategies

You must generate a list of alternative strategies that will achieve the goals you have established. In accomplishing this activity you will use resources such as your knowledge base and experience, a review of your patient assessment, the knowledge of other members of the health care team, and (time allowing) a review of literature. For each alternative solution on the list, you will want to determine mentally if it is realistic, that is, if it is something that can be accomplished, is cost effective, and is beneficial. You should also consider the consequences. This will allow you to predict which alternative(s) will most likely achieve the desired outcome.

Step 5: Select the Strategy

In step 5 of the decision-making process, you will pull together all the information gathered previously to select the best strategy. As you did in prioritizing goals in step 3, you will place your alternatives in rank order, according to how well you believe they will achieve your goals.

At this point we need a system that will allow us to weigh the various aspects and determine the overall value of each strategy (possible solution) that has been identified. Theoretically at least, the alternative with the highest value will be the one selected, implemented, and evaluated. You can attach a weighted value to each possible strategy using a numerical scoring tool that will be discussed later in this chapter. Essentially, you would assign one score ranging from 1 to 10 that is based on the possibility of achieving the result. You would assign a second score based on the desirability of the action. Other factors, such as cost or time, might also be assigned scores. These scores would then be totaled and the total score could be used to rank the possible strategies. When you have made your choice on which alternative strategy to implement, you must always be able to provide sound rationale for your decision to others. Interventions without clear, correct, or defensible rationale are dangerous and impede effective decision making (Beyers & Dudas, 1984).

Step 6: Implement the Strategy

Intertwined with the decision of why this intervention strategy should be used are decisions related to how the strategy you have selected will actually be implemented. Johnson and Davis (1975) have included the following in a list of guidelines:

1. List the actions that must be done to prepare for and actually implement the decision.
2. Estimate the knowledge and skills necessary to carry out the actions safely.
3. Identify the health team members who are available and possess the necessary knowledge and skills.
4. Determine the time, equipment, and supplies needed to implement the action(s).
5. Prioritize related or multiple actions.
6. Communicate this information to other members of the health care team.

Nurses must make many decisions. It is not necessary or appropriate that they personally implement all the decisions. You may implement the decision; or prepare, direct, and supervise others as they implement it. Deciding who should implement the decision is important. Some will be implemented best by the nurse; others may be implemented by another health care worker. In either case, as the decision maker you have the responsibility and accountability for the outcome.

Because you have the responsibility and accountability for the action decided upon, you will want to maintain a suitable amount of control over the implementation. Sound communication skills will facilitate this. You will want to be clear and specific about your decision, what you want to have done, what reports you expect to receive, and when you expect actions to be completed. You will want to verify that your message was correctly understood and you will want to do a systematic followup to determine that all went as planned. Proper implementation plays a critical role in assuring that the decision making was effective.

Step 7: Evaluate

Evaluation is the final step in the decision-making process. You will compare the current situation to the original condition and to the ideal situation. You know that the decision-making process was effective when the current situation matches or is close to the desired situation. The decision was ineffective if the current situation is very little better (or perhaps worse) than the original situation.

To assure maximum objectivity in the evaluation process, you will look at the current situation (outcome) in relation to specific and measurable short-term goals. When properly stated, goals are objective and measurable. Many can be evaluated with a simple yes or no.

When you have determined that your decision was effective, you should review the process. This allows you to review the situation for new problems. It also helps you to identify those steps that worked for you so that you may use them in future decision making.

What do you do if, in the evaluation process, you realize your decision making has been ineffective? You begin by reviewing the seven steps just outlined. It is possible that one or more of the following errors occurred:

- Assessment data were erroneous and/or incomplete.
- Assessment data were improperly analyzed.
- Problems were not correctly identified.
- Problems were not appropriately prioritized.
- Goals were unrealistic or unfeasible.
- Decisions were reached without knowledge and analysis of all possible alternatives and possible consequences.
- Decisions were incorrectly implemented.
- Evaluation of responses (outcomes) was incomplete.
- The decision maker had limited knowledge or experience with which to make the decision.
- The situation changed so rapidly that it was not possible to act quickly enough.

TERMS RELEVANT TO DECISION MAKING

In the list we just provided and occasionally throughout the discussion of the steps in decision making we used terms such as *responsibility, authority, effective, ineffective, feasible,* and *realistic.* Let's review what this terminology means when applied to the decision-making process.

Responsibility and Authority

We have talked about the nurse manager as being responsible for making effective decisions. *Responsibility* means being held accountable for something. The nurse manager is responsible for making decisions that promote quality patient care. This manager is accountable first and foremost to the patient, then to other members of the health care team, to the administrators of the care facility, to the discipline of nursing, and to society as a whole. The nurse is accountable not only for decisions but for the consequences of those decisions (Beyers & Dudas, 1984).

As noted at the beginning of this chapter, nurses always have had a lot of responsibility, but until recently they have not always had appropriate authority to accompany it. *Authority* is the power or the right to give commands, enforce obedience, take action, or make final decisions. Authority is used to fulfill responsibilities. Increasingly nurses are being given authority commensurate with their degree of responsibility and education. Goodman (1965) states that the best decision making involves at the level of action the persons most prepared to make the decisions, those responsible for making decisions, those constantly in the situation. Applying this to the patient care environment, it is the nurse who has the necessary preparation, responsibility, and constant contact required for making effective decisions.

Effective and Ineffective Decisions

Effective decisions meet or come close to meeting the goals that were established in the decision-making process. Critical to this process is preparing goals and objectives that are specific and measurable (see Chap. 3). Ineffective decisions, on the other hand, would be those that do not meet the established goals and objectives.

Realistic and Feasible Decisions

The terms *realistic* and *feasible* are important when discussing decision making. A *realistic* decision is one that is physically possible or that fits the circumstances or situation. For example, if you decide a hospitalized bilateral amputee is to engage in ambulation in order to prevent pneumonia, your decision is not realistic. For this patient it would be more realistic to speak to the physician concerning respiratory care treatments to prevent pneumonia.

A *feasible* decision is one that it is possible to carry out in light of the resources available in the patient care environment. For example, if you decide that an older adult patient would benefit from a bedside commode and no bedside commode is available within your facility, your decision is not feasible.

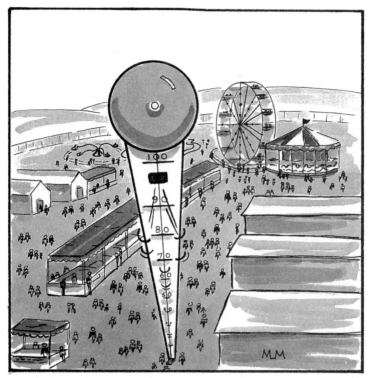

Effective decisions are those that meet or come close to meeting the goals that were established.

FORMAL APPROACHES TO DECISION MAKING

Nurses can use many approaches to assist in consistently making effective decisions. Most of these approaches can be employed either as an individual making the decision or as a member of a group responsible for making the decision.

Listing Pros and Cons

Everyone is familiar with the process of listing pros and cons, having used it to assist with everyday decisions. It involves listing the pros (the advantages or favorable consequences of an action or strategy) and the cons (the disadvantages or unfavorable consequences). With this approach the nurse must know the various alternatives and the general pros and cons of each (Alfaro, 1986). Armed with this information, the nurse then analyzes each alternative with regard to the specific situation and writes a list of specific pros and cons for the strategy. Typically, the strategy chosen for implementation is that with the longest list of pros and the shortest list of cons. The strategy might also be evaluated from the perspective of which is most beneficial or least harmful.

The advantages of listing pros and cons are that listing is simple, is direct, and can be done quickly. The disadvantage is that it is difficult to know all the possible alternative strategies and their various pros and cons in a typically brief time. There may also be overreliance on both the subjective aspects of each pro or con and the number of pros versus the number of cons. Additionally, no method will allow you to compare and contrast objectively the various alternatives. Nurses frequently use this approach for problems requiring an immediate decision and where the focus is short term.

Decision Trees

Another aid to decision making is the use of decision trees. A decision tree is a graphic tool that allows the nurse manager to identify the alternative solutions, to see what factors need to be considered, and to look at the probable outcomes. The manager is given all the pertinent data, which are then plotted on a tree. Each alternative or strategy is plotted as a branch on the tree, which is then divided into subbranches that identify critical factors to consider. Risk factors can also be added. The size of the tree and the number of branches on the tree depend on the resources and number of persons involved and on how critical the decision may be. Establishing decision trees helps us to identify possible alternatives and to approach the decision-making process with more information. It allows us to break down complex decisions into a series of smaller decisions and to illustrate the components of the larger decision. An example of a decision tree for pressure ulcers is provided in Figure 6–1. Decision trees also have their limitations. They assume that all alternatives involved in the decision (the branches on the tree) are known, clearly definable, mutually exclusive, and time-sequenced. In the typical patient care environment, we rarely know all the possible aspects of a situation. Even if we had all this information, the decision tree might become so large and congested it would be confusing and would no longer assist in decision making.

The Matrix or Decision Grid

The matrix or decision grid involves a visual grid that allows us to compare alternative strategies for attacking an actual or potential problem. Various factors relevant to the decision, such as cost, time, and resources, are written across the top of the grid. The alternative strategies are listed down the side of the grid. Decision grids are more graphic and more complete than listing pros and cons, in that they expand the list of pros and cons. Because decision grids are generally less complex than decision tress, they are frequently used as complements to decision trees (Prescott, Dennis & Jacox, 1987).

Numerical Scoring

The process for numerical scoring was discussed earlier in this chapter; therefore, it requires only a brief review here. As described earlier, this system allows us to weight the relative merit of alternative strategies. Each aspect of the situation is subjectively considered and assigned a numerical value. Scores may be assigned for desirability, possibility of success, and other factors, such as cost and time. These are then totaled and a decision is reached based upon the score.

Numerical scoring has the advantage of being relatively simple. It forces the decision maker to write things down and to look at alternatives. It facilitates reanalysis and allows for the simultaneous and systematic consideration of more than one alternative with minimal confusion.

The disadvantage of numerical scoring is that the valuation and assignment of numbers are somewhat arbitrary and subjective. However, it is a skill that can be learned and developed.

PARTICIPATIVE DECISION MAKING

With the advent of less authoritarian approaches to management and with shared governance becoming more and more popular, participative techniques to decision making have received more attention. Participative decision making means allowing a group of individuals to make the decision rather than a single individual. Several different processes are currently being used. We will discuss some of the more commonly used approaches.

The Task Force

A task force is frequently used to address a single problem or concern. A relatively inexpensive technique, it begins with the manager appointing a group of individuals to work on the specific problem. They collect information, analyze it, outline alternatives, make a recommendation, and send that recommendation to the manager. They are then adjourned and do not reconvene unless requested to do so. You can see that one of the major attributes of this process is its ability to capitalize on the expertise of members of the task force.

(*Text continues on page 134*)

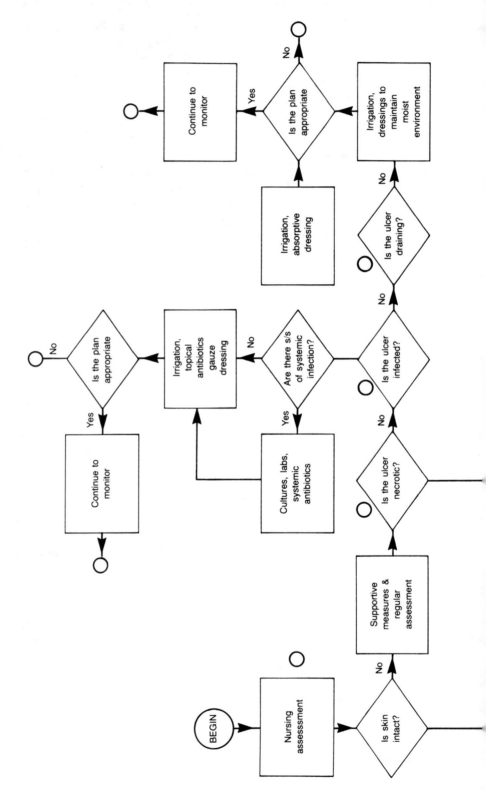

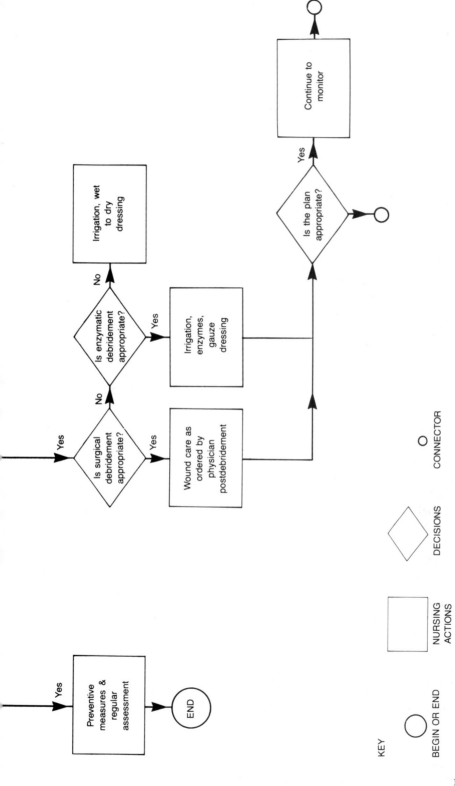

Figure 6-1. Example of a decision tree dealing with pressure ulcers.

133

Quality Circles

Quality circles function much like task forces, with the exception that the membership is usually on a volunteer rather than an appointment basis, and the membership may rotate. Quality circles tend to bring together persons working in the same area who have common concerns. They meet on a regular basis to creatively address day-to-day problems.

Brainstorming

Brainstorming is a fairly expensive process and may have been overused in the last decade. The manager plans a "retreat" away from the work environment at which participants think "freely" of all possible solutions. All ideas brought forth are considered worthy of further review. It is believed that when the participants are away from the constraints of the work environment, such as telephone interruptions and other activities, better ideas will be generated. A "good" brainstorming session may last 2 or 3 days.

There has been a tendency to lapse into a "brainstorming" method of solving problems in the work environment. A manager, when meeting with the staff, will say, "Let's brainstorm that problem for awhile." This negates some of the positive attributes of the process, because the focus of the meeting and its setting will limit the creativity put forth.

Nominal Group Technique

The nominal group technique involves 7 to 10 individuals selected by the manager. The manager presents the problem to the group and each participant writes down what he or she sees as the best solution without discussing it with others. These ideas are then shared with the group and are written on a chalkboard or flip chart. There is no discussion until all ideas are written down. Then each solution is analyzed in light of the problem and participants are asked to rank the solutions privately and individually from most acceptable to least acceptable. The solution that receives the highest overall ranking is then presented as the first alternative. This process allows for consideration of a number of approaches without the members of the group being pressured toward a particular approach.

The Delphi Method

The Delphi method is similar to that of the nominal group technique. All information is gathered about the problems, solutions are outlined, and all possible solutions are shared with the participants who select the best

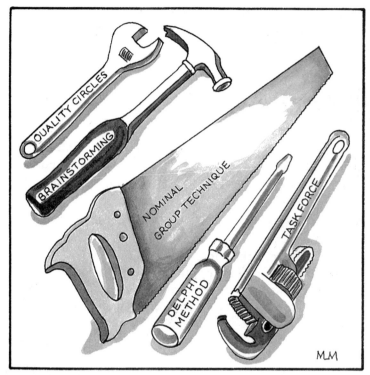

A number of tools can assist in the process of participative decision making.

alternative. However, the membership of the group is anonymous, with only the manager knowing to whom he has sent information and/or questionnaires. This completely prevents one person influencing the decision of another. Because the participants are never identified by name, they are free to approach the problem objectively without fear of repercussions.

CHARACTERISTICS OF THE EFFECTIVE DECISION MAKER

Many personal characteristics affect a nurse's ability to make effective decisions. The nurse's own philosophy, beliefs, and knowledge about nursing, human beings, and health care influence what and how decisions are made. The ability of the nurse to communicate and reason also affects the decision-making process.

The nurse who consistently makes effective decisions develops and maintains a current knowledge base. Active participation in continuing education programs coupled with ongoing self-study and clinical experience are hallmarks of the career nurse who makes good decisions (Aspinall & Tanner, 1981).

GUIDELINES FOR DECISION MAKING

Using a systematic, comprehensive approach to decision making is the secret of consistently arriving at a decision that will have positive outcomes. In addition, we offer the following suggestions regarding the process:

- Always consider the time element involved in reaching the decision. Some decisions must be made in seconds, whereas others may require weeks of deliberation.
- Use the full period of time you have available for the process. Do not rush yourself, but at the same time, do not dawdle.
- Once you have made the decision, implement it as quickly as the situation will allow.
- Always be clear about the situation. Have firsthand knowledge at your fingertips at all times.
- Stay current with regard to your knowledge of nursing, patient care, and the patient care environment.
- Communicate frequently and effectively with others.

SUMMARY

Effective decision making is best approached in a systematic and comprehensive manner. Critical to the process is the nurse's prior knowledge about health care, clinical experience, and practice in decision making. Decision making involves a seven-step process that includes assessing the situation, defining the problem, determining short- and long-term goals, analyzing alternatives, selecting a strategy, implementing the strategy, and evaluating the outcome. Effective decision making requires that the decisions be realistic and feasible and that the nurse have appropriate authority to match the responsibility and accountability demanded in the decision-making process.

A number of tools or aids to the decision-making process are available. These include listing pros and cons; using decision trees, decision grids, or matrixes; and weighing alternatives with a numerical scoring system.

Participatory decision making is commonly employed in today's society. Some techniques for participatory decision making include the use of a task force or quality circles, brainstorming, nominal group techniques, and the Delphi method.

The knowledgeable nurse makes consistently good decisions. In reaching these decisions the nurse considers the time allowed and the situation. The nurse promptly implements the decision reached and uses good communication skills to assure that the decision is appropriately implemented and evaluated.

Study Questions/Activities

1. What is the challenge to nurses?
2. List and describe effective decisions you have made in the clinical setting.
3. What process did you use to make those decisions?
4. Compare and contrast your method(s) for decision making with the overall process for effective decision making outlined in this chapter.
5. In relation to a particular decision in a patient care environment with which you are familiar, describe how you would use the various approaches and tools for effective decision making outlined in this chapter.
6. What tips could you offer on how to make effective decisions consistently?

REFERENCES

Alfaro, R. (1986). *Application of nursing process: A step by step guide.* Philadelphia: J.B. Lippincott.

Aspinall, M., & Tanner, C. (1981). *Decision-making for patient care: Applying the nursing process.* New York: Appleton-Century-Crofts.

Bailey, J., & Claus, K. (1975). *Decision making in nursing: Tools for change.* St. Louis: C.V. Mosby.

Barry, P. (1989). *Psychosocial nursing: Assessment and intervention.* Philadelphia: J.B. Lippincott.

Beyers, M. & Dudas, S. (1984). *The clinical practice of medical–surgical nursing.* Boston: Little, Brown & Co.

Duespohl, T. (1983). *Nursing in transition.* Rockville, Md.: Aspen Systems.

Goodman, P. (1965). *People or personnel: Decentralization and the mixed system.* New York: Random House.

Johnson, M., & Davis, M. (1975). *Problem solving in nursing practice.* Dubuque, Ia.: Brown.

Lewis, L. (1970). *Planning patient care.* Dubuque, Ia.: Brown.

Matteson, M., & McConnell, E. (1988). *Gerontological nursing: Concepts and practice.* Philadelphia: W.B. Saunders.

Prescott, P., Dennis, K., & Jacox, A. (1987). Clinical decision-making of staff nurses. *Image, 19,* 56–62.

Roemer, M. (1986). *An introduction to the U.S. health care system.* New York: Springer.

SUGGESTIONS FOR FURTHER READING

Albert, D. (1978). Decision theory in medicine: A review and critique. *Milbank Memorial Fund Quarterly: Health and Society, 56,* 362–401.

Freund, C. (1988). Decision making styles. *Journal of Nursing Administration, 18*(12), 5–11.

Fryback, D. (1981). A note about decision trees. In M. Aspinall & C. Tanner, *Decision-making for patient care: Applying the nursing process.* New York: Appleton-Century-Crofts (pp. 349–352).

Joiner, C., & Corkrean, M. (1986). *Critical incidents in nursing management.* Norwalk, Conn.: Appleton-Century-Crofts.

Kepner, C., & Tregoe, B. (1985). *The rational manager.* New York: McGraw-Hill.

Matheson, J., & Howard, R. (1976). An introduction to decision analysis. In R. Howard, J. Matheson, & K. Miller (Eds.), *Readings in decision analysis.* Menlo Park, Calif.: Stanford Research Institute.

Smith, A. (1982). *Management systems: Analyses and applications.* New York: CBS College Publishing.

Managing Time Effectively

7

Objectives

After completing this chapter, you should be able to:

1. *Increase awareness of how your time is managed.*
2. *Recognize personal and professional "time wasters" and "time savers."*
3. *Incorporate techniques that can be used for better personal and professional time management.*
4. *Understand the importance of leisure when structuring time.*
5. *Apply the various principles of time management in the clinical setting.*

Humans have always had a sense of time, even when precise measurement was impossible. Our bodies tell us daily of the passing of time by an awareness of our unique but subtle body rhythms. We know when we are hungry, when we are sleepy. In a more extended way, we know time is passing by visible signs of aging; wrinkles and gray hair appear. Older cultures, unencumbered by clocks and calendars, marked time by recording the movement of the sun, the position of the stars, and the passing of seasons.

The first clock was reported to have been designed in the ninth century, but it was some time before people owned their own timepieces. Early European clocks of the eleventh and twelfth centuries were installed in church towers only to call worshipers to prayer. People did not have personal timepieces. Since that time, modern society has treated the clock as a necessity. Homes and workplaces often have more than one clock, and it is unusual to find people who do not wear wristwatches. Some people on holiday may remove their watches in an attempt to separate themselves from the time demands of work and home. Scientific clocks have achieved nearly perfect measurement of time.

Several factors affect how each of us views and manages time in everyday life. If we come from a culture in which time is seen as less rigid than in Western society, it may be very difficult to adjust to the ever-present time demands of family, school, and work. Western cultures are not as forgiving of tardiness as are some other cultures. Another factor affecting the way we view time is the way the family in which we grew up viewed it. For example, if your parent or parents worked a 9 A.M. to 5 P.M. day and dinner was always served sharply at 6 P.M., as an adult you may need to carry on your life with strict time lines; or you may decide that time demands were a burden and purposely structure your life around more relaxed time frames.

Aside from both culture and family style, psychological status also contributes to how time is viewed. People experiencing normal grief reactions often have time distortion. Studies have shown that clergy and funeral directors frequently find that survivors are either early or late for appointments or may not even appear because of their emotional distress. More generally, insecurity may produce an increased need for the psychological comfort provided by rigid time management. Time requirements can serve as a method for limit setting. For example, clearly set time expectations may be comfortable for people because decisions have already been made about how time is to be spent. Other persons may rebel against time requirements that they view as being imposed on them by others and may react by ignoring time requirements altogether.

The increased sophistication of time measurement has paralleled our interest and even obsession with time. We have become, in large part, a time-oriented society. "Faster is better!" Getting more done is rewarded. Time management often guides our perceptions of others and of ourselves. How we manage time can make us feel good and confident about ourselves or make us feel inadequate. Time management may play a large part in whether we get a coveted job or lose it.

Industry has recognized the economic value of time management for a long time. If workers manage time well, production increases. Corporations have spent large sums of money holding seminars for management and workers relating to time management. Time saved is money saved (Table 7–1). Rifkin states, "It is ironic in a culture so committed to saving time we feel increasingly deprived of the very thing we value. What time we do have is chopped up into tiny segments, each filled in with prior commitments and plans. Our tomorrows are spoken for, booked up in advance. We rarely have a moment to spare" (1987, p. 11). It should not surprise us that time management is closely linked to stress management. Many of our everyday stresses are a direct result of the "time crunch" in which we find ourselves.

It is important to mention the existence of the "workaholic" personality. Workaholics may or may not use time wisely, but they are only comfortable when constantly "doing" things. They feel guilt if they are not working, and they cannot enjoy leisure. These persons often have physical and emotional problems resulting from this behavior. The primary reason for our considering the many time management techniques in this chapter is to get more done in less time, so that we are more free to enjoy time for ourselves and those important to us.

TABLE 7–1. THE VALUE OF YOUR TIME (in dollars)

Annual Earnings	Worth per Hour	Worth per Minute	Worth in One Year if You Saved 1 Hour Each Day
$ 5,000	$ 2.56	$0.043	$ 625
10,000	5.12	0.085	1250
15,000	7.68	0.123	1875
20,000	10.25	0.131	2500
25,000	12.81	0.219	3125
30,000	15.37	0.256	3750
35,000	17.93	0.299	4375
40,000	20.49	0.341	5000
45,000	23.05	0.384	5625
50,000	25.61	0.427	6250

LEARNING TO MANAGE TIME

At first, going through the steps necessary for establishing better time management may seem difficult and actually wasteful of time that could be spent in other ways. However, once you have learned actions that may help your personal management of time, you will find it becomes "second nature." You may already be a very good time manager, but everyone can become better; by learning one new action, you may save an undetermined amount of time for other things in your life. Some people report that when they feel time stressed, they revert back to time management principles. Knowing and adopting a time management program, however, help us reduce stress imposed by time constraints, so that more is accomplished in less time. "To manage means to have a system—and it helps if the system works" (Davidson, 1978, p. 13). In this chapter we shall discuss the setting of goals and managing time more effectively, so that you can move toward fulfillment of the goals you have set for yourself. Throughout this chapter you will see how you can apply concepts of time management to your personal life as well as to nursing.

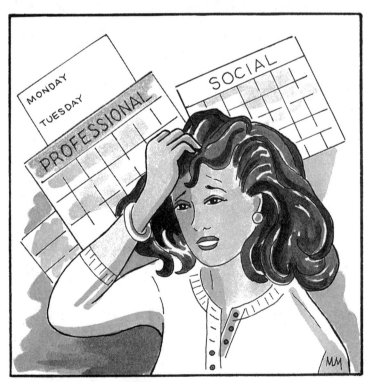

Knowing and adopting a time management program helps reduce stress imposed by time constraints.

BENEFITS OF EFFECTIVE TIME MANAGEMENT

Each of us has only 24 hours, or 1440 minutes, in each day. Finding ways to use this circumscribed time better offers many benefits that may not be obvious. We can gain better control over life, accomplish more in less time, decrease anxiety, increase satisfaction, and provide more leisure time through effective time management.

Perhaps one of the greatest benefits of effectively managing time is that we control time rather than allowing it to control us. Do you control your time or does time control you? In our society, by necessity, some of our time is controlled, but this should be only with our consent. For example, you must be in class at 8:30 in the morning. Because of this, your alarm clock and watch take on increased importance. However, it is ultimately your choice to attend class and be prompt. The consequences of not doing so may not be productive to passing the course. Because one of your goals (discussed next) is to pass the course, your decision to attend class is an action that is necessary but also voluntary on your part.

Many think that time management is about doing more. In fact, if doing more simply means to the individual having more work to do, there may be less desire to change. Time management means gaining maximum return on time invested. Managing time effectively results in taking less time to accomplish tasks. This gives us more time for leisure and other meaningful pursuits in our lives while also accomplishing the tasks of school or work.

Because we can accomplish more in less time with good management, it follows that the energy we put into projects is conserved and that returns are greater on the time we do spend.

Nothing is more anxiety generating than to feel that you are always "running behind" and that there is never enough time for things you would like to do. With more time in our lives, we can reflect on our accomplishments in a more leisurely fashion that leads to a feeling of personal satisfaction.

The intensity of our lives calls for more leisure time as part of a healthier life-style. But how can we find the time for it? Accomplishing more in less time may provide the time to read a book set aside too long or to listen to a favorite concert. Leisure enhances productivity during the other hours of the day. Lakein writes that "if you arrange things so that you find time to relax and 'do nothing,' you will get more done and have more fun doing it"(1973, p. 53). Daily and weekly leisure combined with family and work result in a more balanced life. Good time management allows and even mandates planning for relaxation.

An additional incentive for individuals who acquire good time management skills is that they tend to manage time in their personal lives as

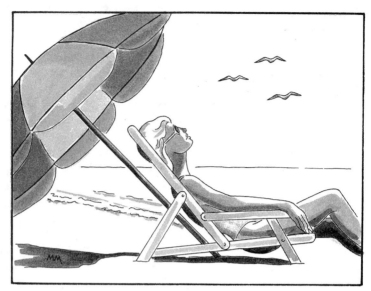

Use of time management techniques allows more free time for leisure.

well as they do in school or the workplace. People may relax using time management principles when there are fewer time demands but revert back to their use when time demands increase.

APPLICATION OF TIME MANAGEMENT TO NURSING

It is curious that time management techniques have largely been directed toward managers within corporations and only recently toward nurse managers. Although managing time is important to the nurse manager, it is as important to everyone on the health care team. Staff nurses and nursing students live very busy lives and must delicately balance their expenditure of time if they are to maintain quality in their daily lives and avoid "burnout" and crumbling relationships.

As you move through this chapter, the application of time management to nursing is clear in that you can use each step as effectively in nursing as you do in personal planning. These techniques are also time savers that are appropriate to a student in a nursing program or a nurse in the clinical setting.

SETTING GOALS

Most people have goals in life but rarely take the time to examine and review them critically. Goals should be written, because writing them down makes them more concrete (Lakein, 1973, p. 31) and forces us to measure them for relevance to our present situation. On a piece of paper take a few minutes and write down your goals. These can be revised later. Goals should be both long and short term, professional and personal. They should be reviewed at least every 3 months and changed if the circumstances in our lives have also changed. Lakein suggests that a "good time to review your goals, particularly lifetime goals is on your birthday" (1973, p. 36). You must also prioritize your goals, so that you clearly see which ones are most important. Two goals can be equally important, such as school and family. These are interrelated, and both goals can be planned for equally.

Goal setting gives you direction for moving into action in order to accomplish what is important to you. Having goals increases confidence, for we see what we really want from life. When goals are fulfilled, we sense satisfaction in moving on to other aspects of our lives. For example, when you complete school, there is tangible evidence that you have attained a goal. A new and exciting goal now becomes success in the workplace.

Write your professional goals. A short-term goal may be that you would like to become a charge nurse on your unit. To accomplish this, your performance and leadership skills will have to be recognized by your supervisor. You may have the long-term goal of acquiring a higher nursing degree. To implement this goal, you will need to save money for tuition and obtain the information provided by nursing schools before you choose your program.

Goals are also important for time management of your work as a nurse. What are the patient's goals and your goals in providing care? You may wish to write these in the goal section on the patient's care plan, or you may choose to write your own informal plan of care that includes goals for an individual patient. Sometimes it is useful to sit quietly the day after your care has been completed for a patient and review your goals for that individual. Reflect then on the nursing actions that will help move that patient toward that goal. For example, if you have a patient with activity intolerance and your goal is to increase activity, you will plan actions that will assist that person toward that goal. If you walked the patient halfway down the corridor today, you may plan to walk the patient the entire length of the corridor tomorrow. You have planned actions that will take time and for which planning is essential to fulfill this goal. The example just given emphasizes that keeping goals manageable and realistic helps when planning care.

Keep in mind that it is important to distinguish between patient goals and nurse goals. At times these may be different. For example, the patient's goal may be to eat and not feel nauseated. Maintaining comfort while eating is a goal for the patient. You understand that this is an important goal for the patient, but it is also your goal to maintain adequate nutrition for the patient.

TIME ASSESSMENT

An interesting and essential first step in beginning to manage time more effectively is to identify how you use time. Only through examining how you spend your time can you begin to set priorities, eliminate time barriers, and incorporate aids to better time management. Most people are surprised by the time assessment exercise, because they have never looked closely at 1 or more days to determine time expenditure. You may know that you are a "morning" or "evening" person, that is, at which time your energy is highest, because you get more done during these hours. A few persons are able to maintain a high energy level consistently throughout the day. Your time assessment chart should validate for you when your energy level is highest or suggest that you are not using your high-energy hours wisely. Consequently, your time assessment chart may direct you to your high-energy times, when it is best to work on projects.

Through assessment you may find that you manage your time very well, but there may be a time waster of which you are not aware. Some find that there are obvious time wasters that can be eliminated. It is also important to recognize your particular time savers. These are behaviors that are sometimes simple but that collectively save time. For example, you might routinely sit down after you return home from school to read the evening paper. For someone living alone, stacking the paper as it is read and picking it up for disposal immediately after reading it means not having to do this later. Admittedly, this may save only a minute or two each day, but this small time saver adds up and results in a neater household.

Using a format similar to that of Table 7–2, list on the right side of the page by the quarter hour exactly how you spent your time. Try to keep the form up to date as you move through each day, because accuracy in recording decreases as you become distracted with the next activity. It is more useful to chart 3 weekdays, because these are usually your busiest days. You may wish to vary the form. For example, if you study in the evening or have an evening class or hospital clinical, you may wish to extend the assessment time into the evening hours. This information is only for your use, and it is not necessary to share it with others unless you wish to do so.

To focus more closely on how you spend your time on the nursing unit, you may do a time assessment of your work hours only. This exercise often proves revealing. For example, if you are on a nursing unit where a good friend is also a staff person, you may not realize the time

TABLE 7-2. TIME ASSESSMENT

Day 1	Day 2	Day 3
6:00	6:00	6:00
6:15	6:15	6:15
6:30	6:30	6:30
6:45	6:45	6:45
7:00	7:00	7:00
7:15	7:15	7:15
7:30	7:30	7:30
7:45	7:45	7:45
8:00	8:00	8:00
8:15	8:15	8:15
8:30	8:30	8:30
8:45	8:45	8:45
9:00	9:00	9:00
9:15	9:15	9:15
9:30	9:30	9:30
9:45	9:45	9:45
10:00	10:00	10:00
10:15	10:15	10:15
10:30	10:30	10:30
10:45	10:45	10:45
11:00	11:00	11:00
11:15	11:15	11:15
11:30	11:30	11:30
11:45	11:45	11:45
12:00	12:00	12:00
12:15	12:15	12:15
12:30	12:30	12:30
12:45	12:45	12:45
1:00	1:00	1:00
1:15	1:15	1:15
1:30	1:30	1:30
1:45	1:45	1:45
2:00	2:00	2:00
2:15	2:15	2:15
2:30	2:30	2:30
2:45	2:45	2:45
3:00	3:00	3:00
3:15	3:15	3:15
3:30	3:30	3:30
3:45	3:45	3:45
4:00	4:00	4:00
4:15	4:15	4:15
4:30	4:30	4:30
4:45	4:45	4:45
5:00	5:00	5:00

Continue on into late afternoon or evening

spent socializing. Perhaps your assessment will show that you spend unnecessary time on the phone, making calls that could appropriately be delegated. Delegation is an important technique we will discuss in more detail later in the chapter.

Looking at both your personal and work time assessment, identify your time wasters as well as your time savers. You may find that there are remarkable similarities between the two, or you may find that you can improve your time management in one area by using techniques that have proved helpful in the other.

TIME MANAGEMENT TECHNIQUES

A Calendar

The selection of a calendar is a very individual pursuit. You probably already have a calendar, but it may not be as useful and functional as you would wish. First, some people find it is most useful to have only *one* calendar. Transferring dates and commitments from one calendar to another is time-consuming. Other people never become comfortable with having only one calendar and prefer to have two. When a single calendar is desired, it should be one that can be carried in either a pocket or a purse. This makes the calendar available for additions and revisions at any given moment. If you have only one calendar, you might wish to photocopy one or more calendar pages from time to time in case the calendar is lost.

Although it is most convenient to have only one calendar, if your professional events and items that need special noting are numerous or complex, you may wish to have a second calendar for professional commitments. If you choose to do this, you must be well organized, so that you either carry both with you at all times, so that you can make notations when you think of them, or leave both in a safe place. Either way it is difficult to avoid becoming confused by utilizing multiple calendars. You are the only one who can determine what works best for you.

Note dates on the calendar in a way that you clearly understand. There is nothing so frustrating as to read a notation you have written quickly or so briefly that you cannot later recall its meaning. For example, you have written, "Dinner with J." Now you wonder: Who is "J"? Where was dinner to be? At what time? You might wish to use symbols such as stars or circles to note certain important dates, such as when papers are due or when a family member will be celebrating an anniversary.

The Tickler File

The term *tickler file* has been in common use for a long time, although its origin is unknown. Tickler files are very helpful in preventing the omission of important dates from the calendar. In essence, this is a reminder list that can be referred to from time to time, so that you will not miss putting important deadlines and dates on your daily calendar. You can effectively use tickler files by listing the important requirements of the quarter or semester. You might note when papers and other assignments are due. Using this method, you would know when several assignments are due within a short time. Start and stop dates for classes and clinical experiences can also be listed in the file. As a staff nurse, you can also use a tickler file to remember important dates that are pending. Examples are clinical care conferences or classes in your area of practice.

Personal items can be included. Perhaps you are to make a dentist appointment in 2 months. A short note about this would remind you in time to make arrangements. A future wedding could also be noted. Tickler files save time by highlighting future important events.

Making a "To Do" List

A daily "to do" list is a necessary aid when establishing priorities as well as for determining what is to be done each day. A "to do" list should not be limited to work items but should also include time for leisure.

The time assessment exercise you have done may lead you to conclude that you have been unrealistic in the number of tasks you attempted in a given day and that you are now ready to write a more realistic plan. The "to do" list could be compared to a grocery shopping list. It is curious that many people would not think of entering a grocery store without a list of items to be purchased and yet postpone or avoid making a list of activities to be accomplished in the period of that day or the day following.

Whether a "to do" list is made in the evening or morning is not as important as consistently making out such a list in written form. The time chosen for beginning such a list is very individual. Some complete the day by thinking about what should be done tomorrow. Others, often early risers, prefer to sit quietly in the morning and look at the day before them and decide what must be done. It is best simply to list tasks. You may find it helpful to keep a "running list," adding to it as you think of additional tasks. Prioritizing tasks will be the next step. See Table 7–3 for an example of a personal "to do" list that has been prioritized.

A "to do" list will be especially important when as a charge nurse or manager you are responsible for the work of others as well as your own. Your list might contain tasks of others that you need to double-check. For example, you might need to check whether the student nurse has com-

TABLE 7–3. A PERSONAL PRIORITIZED "To Do" LIST AND DELEGATED TASKS

Pick up dry cleaning	C
Visit Joan's teacher at school @ 2 P.M.	A
Study for Friday quiz	A
Bake cookies for Joan's class (party tomorrow)	A (d)
Change sheets on beds	C (B)
Shop for weekend	C (B)
Get tire replaced/new on right rear	A
Call for dentist appt.	C
Order bulbs from catalog .	C
Time with Joan	A
Buy text for fall quarter	C
Drop off plant food at Mother's	B (A)
Dust	B (A) (d)
Fix dinner—casserole (?)	A
Check batteries in smoke alarm	A
Sew button on winter coat	C (d)
Lecture class (2 hours)	A
Buy surprise for Joan	A
Sort through winter clothes/discard	C
Write letter to Uncle Ray	B (C)
Sort mail	B (A)
Pay bills	B (C)
Walk dog	A (d)
Buy dog food at pet shop	B (A)
Call church choir members	C (d)

Delegated Tasks	To Whom
Bake cookies	Joan or mother
Dust	Joan
Sew on button	mother
Walk dog	Joan
Call church choir	Choir vice-pres

★ d = delegate

pleted the pain management flow sheet correctly. It might include tasks that affect the work of others, such as contacting a physician for an order for bowel care that will be done by the licensed practical nurse. By writing these items down you are less likely to forget something important. After you have written your list, you can refine and prioritize the items on it using the following techniques. Without priorities you may run out of time before an important task is done or you may not attend to a task that needs prompt attention.

Prioritizing the "To Do" List

Your list may contain far too many activities to be accomplished in the time available. Not all items on a list are equally important. Some items should not wait. Lakein has devised a very helpful method of prioritizing tasks. He states, "What is the best use of my time right now?" (1973, p. 7). At 9 o'clock in the morning, the answer for you may be reading the assigned material for the 1-o'clock lecture. This item will be designated an A item. Fixing or replacing a defective automobile tire concerns safety and perhaps should not be delayed. Therefore, this task will become an A. There may be other A items, things that are time-bound and cannot be put off. Studying for a quiz or writing an assignment are examples of academic tasks that are A's. You will note in Table 7–3 that there are also personal tasks that are A's. Spending time with children or family is important and should be treated as an A.

B's are those tasks that are important but not urgent. One of the B tasks in Table 7–3 might be calling for a routine dentist appointment. This is important but need not be done on a particularly busy day. Tasks designated as C are neither as important nor as urgent as A or B items. An example of a C task in Table 7–3 is "sort through winter clothes and discard." Because the date of the list is mid-April, this could wait until summer break. It is not a priority at this time.

After you have listed the tasks, it is helpful to look over the list and see if there are any items that can be delegated to someone else. This may shorten the list considerably. We shall talk more about delegation a little later in the chapter, but for now, look back at Table 7–3. Although it is a hypothetical list, Joan, the daughter, may be old enough to take on some of the tasks. She may do the dusting, change the sheets on the bed, or even bake the cookies.

When you have decided which items on your "to do" list can be delegated and which are A's, B's, or C's, go back and place the B items in either the A or C category. This practice forces us to prioritize and therefore produces a workable list for the next day. You will notice that the B tasks in Table 7–3 have been changed to either A or C.

You can then arrange your daily schedule to include both A and C items. If possible, arrange your schedule to work on A items during your high-energy-level times and leave C items for times when you have less energy. You can also group tasks together to save both time and energy. Referring back to Table 7–3, you could visit Joan's class at school before dropping off plant food at your mother's. You might even wish to take your winter coat and the detached button for her to sew. The pet shop stop is very time-consuming, so that picking up pet food at the same place you usually shop could be a positive option.

The professional "to do" list that you prepare for patient care also helps structure your workday (see Table 7–4). It helps identify the best use of your time with patients. This list cannot be rigid. Flexibility in caring for patients is essential, for many events may require you to change

TABLE 7–4. A PROFESSIONAL PRIORITIZED "To Do" LIST AND DELEGATED TASKS

Mr. Audrey:	
Look for lost hearing aid	C (A)
Post notice so he gets morning paper	B (A) (d)
Range of motion × 3 (adding one)	A
Explain call light system again	A
Ask family to bring in radio	B (C) (d)
Mrs. Shelton:	
Finish care plan	A
Find out policy on visiting by 4-year-old daughter	B (A)
Assist in walking 2 × per shift	A
Order egg crate mattress	A (d)
Notify dietitian of milk intolerance	A (d)
Miss Davies:	
Check on telephone repair	A (d)
Call Social Service regarding discharge	A
Telephone clergy office and ask for visit	C (A) (d)
Personal:	
See unit manager regarding date for evlauation conference	C
Ask for a locker closer to top of cabinet	C
See schedule for Memorial Day holiday	A
Put in request for summer vacation in July	B (C)

Delegated Tasks	**To Whom**
Mr. Audrey:	
Morning paper notice	Nursing assistant
Call family for radio	Nursing assistant or unit secretary
Mrs. Shelton:	
Order egg crate mattress	Unit secretary
Phone dietitian to report pt. milk intolerance	Nursing assistant
Miss Davies:	
Telephone repair	Unit secretary
Clergy consult	Nursing assistant

★ d = delegate

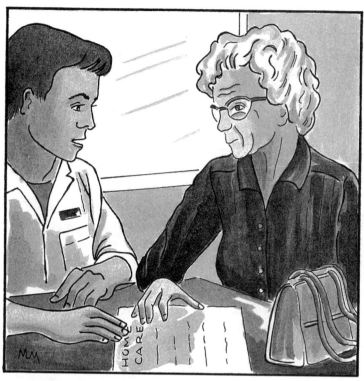

A "to do" list such as you use to structure your own workday may help a patient plan for home care.

your plans. However, you can set priorities. Which of these actions is the most important for the patient's care? Which are the C items, those you would like to implement but that are not crucial to health or safety? A situation that often arises is that the unit is short of staff, forcing you to concentrate on A items for the day and either delegate or delay actions that you have deemed C. You will find that delegating and rearranging your "to do" list as you plan your day often makes what appeared to be an unrealistic schedule manageable.

AIDS TO TIME MANAGEMENT

There are a variety of strategies to better manage your time. Let us consider some of the more important ones that can be used in either your personal life or your nursing career.

Writing Things Down

Although most of us think that we have a very good memory, it is more efficient and time-saving to develop the habit of writing things down. You should have a special place to write down things other than on your "to do" list. Persons who manage time effectively sometimes carry 3 × 5 blank cards in a purse or pocket. A supply of these cards could also be kept in your car or at your bedside in case you think of something before retiring or during the night. Writing down your thoughts about projects or things to do relieves your mind and you can use your energy on getting things done rather than on trying to remember what it was that you had in mind. Commercially made "sticky notes" have been valuable to many people in remembering short-term, nonessential items. You can paste these on your bathroom mirror at home or on your locker at work to remind you visually of something you intend doing.

Learning to Say No

One of the most difficult things for sensitive care providers is to say *no* when asked to do or help with a task. First of all, there are things you may be asked to do that are truly not appropriate—for which you have no skills. It is essential that you honestly recognize these instances and that you decline when they occur. These may be personal or professional events. For example, if your organization asks you to chair a committee whose task is to plan the budget and you know this is an area that you neither enjoy nor have expertise in, it is only fair to everyone to decline. If you are a beginning nursing student on a hospital unit and a staff nurse asks you to observe a very ill patient "only for a few minutes until I get back," you have the obligation to refuse. Not declining could jeopardize the patient's safety.

There may be other times when you are asked to do something enjoyable and yet you realize that your busy schedule will not allow you to take on any additional responsibility. You can be gracious yet realistic and truthful with your reply: "I would really have enjoyed doing this for you, but it is impossible for me to become involved in anything else right now." If you might be available in the future, you could say, "Thank you for asking me, but I can't take this on right now. You might want to ask me again in the summer, when I will have more time."

Before saying no, consider the amount of time you or the person who is asking thinks the request will reasonably take. You may have to ask. Also consider who the person is who is asking you to do something. It may be easier to say no to a telephone request to help with the annual fund drive of a charitable agency than it would be to say no to your instructor, supervisor, or family member. Also, weigh how much you value the activity you are declining. For example, although you would both value and enjoy helping plan the class reunion, you may decline because of time pressures and limit your involvement to only attending the event.

Using Energy Effectively

As we have stated, the time when your energy is highest relates to your specific body rhythms. You may also find that you are not as energetic during times of personal stress or illness. Using your "to do" list, it is generally best to choose your high-energy hours to undertake the A tasks that are most important and difficult. Many nurses choose to implement A nursing actions early in the shift, when energy seems to be highest. If you only have a limited amount of time, you could either do one part of an A task or perform a C task that requires less time. There may be a time when you have a cold or are tired and not feeling energetic. Rather than abandon the entire list, you could work on several C items that are less demanding with a time frame designed to move to A's later.

Finding Privacy

It is essential for you to find some private time each day for reflection, relaxation, or performing important tasks. Webber calls this "isolation" and states that it is important to find a place that affords uninterrupted time (1980, p. 49). Finding such a place is hard for most busy people.

Students, who must study, have particular difficulty finding a location in which they will not be disturbed. When it is feasible, going to the library to study is a good option. The environment of libraries is designed for reading and quiet study. If this is impossible, having a special place in your home is useful. Study materials at home should be moved about as little as possible. Simply closing a door with a short but polite explanation can be effective in separating you from others. Having to clear books and papers away so that family activities can take place and then having to get them out again is very time-consuming. Depending on the individual, certain components seem to optimize the environment for study. For some, music may provide an atmosphere conducive to study; for others it may interfere with concentration. These suggestions can also work well on a nursing unit when you must chart on a record or tape a report. Be sure, however, to check the hospital policy regarding location of records.

Minimizing Interruptions

Interruptions can intrude on privacy, breaking the thought process in such a way that it takes more time to complete a task. Do a quick assessment. What are your primary interruptions? We shall be discussing telephone messages, visitors, and other interruptions later, but one interruption frequently cited by families is that of children.

One parent who was unable to study because of the interruptions imposed by a 4-year-old found a creative solution. At the end of the week she purchased the next week's supply of inexpensive "surprises" at the store. For example, a box of crayons was divided into several packages. When it was time to study, she explained her study needs to the child, set a timer, and closed the door, with the instruction that she was to be in her private place (except for emergencies) until the timer sounded. Then the child would receive a "surprise" and the two would spend some needed time together. (Of course, a very small child should be checked from time to time.) These creative touches are very much a part of managing your time better.

It is often difficult to avoid interruptions on the nursing unit. You may have to be assertive in informing other staff members that you need time alone to perform certain tasks. One of these tasks is the patient's nursing care plan. You can write a more thoughtful plan of care if you are in a quiet place where there are minimum interruptions.

Avoiding Paper Shuffling

Many experts in time management state that a person should only "touch paper once." This principle helps us avoid the time-consuming tendency of stacking papers and notes and then later restacking and reordering them. The paper shuffler is a time waster. Some people avoid proceeding with tasks by feeling that they are doing something by shuffling papers. The technique to avoid shuffling papers takes both practice and restraint on your part. Our society is composed of paper shufflers. We are a paper society, with mailboxes bulging with advertisements and mail order catalogs. Most of the paper we receive is useless and not worth our time to review. Other papers are more valuable.

Work and school papers are important, and a system must be developed so that they are readily available yet do not require sorting. Notebooks, folders, and files are helpful. A more significant time waster is our daily mail. Once mail is collected from the box, it is time-saving to go through it, keeping only those items that need to be opened and that deserve further scrutiny. Immediately throw out those items that will not be read. Mail that carries a bulk postage rate may not be worth your time. Once mail has been placed in a planned location, it should be dealt with only once, that is, disposed of or given a response.

The same principles apply to the amount of paper to which you are exposed in the clinical setting. First, it helps to use either a clipboard or one piece of paper that is organized for purposes of assessment of your patients. It is confusing and time-consuming to carry around more than one piece of paper; if you do, when it is time to chart, you will have to shuffle through various lists and notations to locate the vital signs on one piece of paper, the intake and output on another, and sometimes special concerns on a third. Second, you may want to join the documentation committee of the unit or the facility in order to revise forms so that unnecessary forms are eliminated and redundancy is reduced on the forms being used.

Shopping More Efficiently

Shopping is a personal task, and one that is very energy depleting. We can conserve much of our energy for family and our nursing profession by learning how to shop more effectively.

Shopping in our society has been made much more time efficient by the advent of supermarkets. The availability of items and household necessities cuts down on the time expended if we learn to shop well. What we suggest does not mean that you will always maintain these shopping habits. You will want to choose the technique that works best for you and your family.

During a period when you have more leisure time, it is fun to enter a new store and observe the variety of unfamiliar products and displays. However, this takes time, and when you are time pressured, it is probably best to shop in a store you know. Knowing the location of products is time-saving. Many supermarkets now have a printout listing the items to be found on the various aisles, so that you can quickly complete your shopping list, saving additional time. Although coupons offering a savings on household items are often economical, it takes time to find the store where the product is available. A "sorter" file can be obtained that you can carry in the store, so that if the coupon item is offered, you can quickly find the coupon and use it for the purchase. This avoids having to visit other retail locations to redeem coupons.

Another aid to more efficient shopping is to combine, or "bunch," errands. For example, going to the gasoline station for gas and making a later trip to the grocery wastes time. Combine as many errands as possible in a single trip. This saves not only time but fuel.

Limiting Socializing

Spending time with friends is understandably pleasant. However, socializing must be controlled if we are to accomplish the many tasks of a busy schedule. You must set limits. If you invite friends to your home, clearly state the time you have available. For example, you might offer an invitation saying, "Could you come over for an early lunch on Saturday? I have to study at 2 o'clock but would love to see you until then." This identifies a time limitation that will not be offensive to your friend.

Set time limits for informal visits. Intrusions by door-to-door salespersons should be met politely but accompanied by your refusal to spend time with unwelcome solicitations. Other unexpected visitors should be told that you have only a limited period of time for a visit. If possible, you should avoid having those acquaintances who come for long periods of time come uninvited. If you wish to see them, it is much more profitable if you go to their home. This gives you the prerogative of leaving when you must do so to spend time on other activities.

Nursing is difficult and our social contacts at work are important to job satisfaction and our mental health. We often reflect with colleagues on our perceptions of clinical situations as well as our personal conflicts. However necessary this is, socialization takes time if it is to be successful. When patient care is a priority, you have to limit social contact. When this is the case, you might say, "I've got to get back to work, but let's have coffee after work so we can visit more freely." Good time managers do not ignore the importance of socialization but strike a balance that leaves time for carrying out patient care effectively.

Limiting Phone Calls

For people who enjoy using the telephone socially, the following suggestions may be difficult to implement. First, you must monitor yourself regarding the importance of a call and the amount of time spent on the phone. Endless social calls are time wasters. You can control your own outgoing calls. You can also control the amount of time spent on incoming calls. You could say to a caller, "I'd like to talk longer but I only have a couple of minutes."

Although many people share a dislike of answering devices in the home, they do serve a legitimate purpose. With such a device you can effectively screen out calls, so that you limit the number to which you respond. You can also eliminate subsequent calls on your part by leaving your message on the machines of other people.

Better Use of Waiting Time

Much time in our society is wasted in waiting: waiting in line, waiting for traffic lights, waiting in offices. The magazines offered in offices of doctors and dentists are often interesting, but they are time wasters. You can take a book or a "to do" list to a waiting room, so that valuable time is not wasted. Audio tapes of texts or lectures can be used in cars. Of course, these should not distract the driver.

Delegating

Just as we hesitate to say no when asked to perform a task, we are reluctant to delegate tasks to others. Delegation decreases demands upon our time. Good time managers learn the technique of delegating successfully and appropriately. Murphy states that we have to move through a process of learning to accept the reality and importance of delegation (1984, p. 54).

On the nursing unit, many nurses make telephone calls or perform secretarial duties that could be delegated, because "it is just faster to do it myself." This is not profitable in the long run, because eliciting the help of the unit secretary or other nonnursing personnel frees up the time of the nurse, who is then able to increase time with the patient. Until you are comfortable with this degree of delegation, carefully consider each phone call you make and whether it could have been made by another person on the unit.

The following are the four guidelines of successful delegation: (1) Be able psychologically to "let go" of the task; (2) choose a capable person to whom to delegate; (3) clearly describe what is to be done; and (4) give praise when a task is accomplished. Let us discuss these more fully.

The first is learning to let go of the responsibility of carrying out a task. Performing tasks well adds to our self-esteem, resulting in a feeling of "ownership." Suppose that, as a staff nurse, you lead a patient care meeting each Monday. If you delegate the leading of the meeting to someone else, you have to trust that person and "let go" of the responsibility.

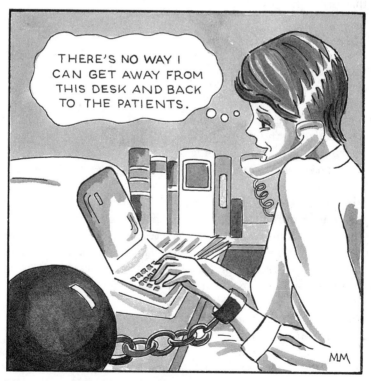

Many nurses make telephone calls or perform secretarial duties that could be delegated.

Letting go of a task is easier if we carefully choose a person who is capable of carrying out the delegated task. The consideration of competency emphasizes the importance of job descriptions. Consider the previous situation of the patient care meeting. If another nurse's job description lists being a backup or substitute for the person regularly leading the conference, then delegation is appropriate. If no other person is designated, a response from the person you ask might have been, "Well, it's not really my job." Always choose someone willing and capable of helping.

Clearly delineate to the person to whom you have delegated the task exactly what is to be done. Clear expectations result in making the person to whom the task was delegated more comfortable.

And finally, when the task has been successfully completed, give recognition and praise for a job well done. If this kind of credit is not forthcoming, it may be difficult for you to find someone to whom you can delegate a job in the future.

A health care team works best when there is mutual delegation. Being a "team player" means that you are considerate of others on the health care team and accept appropriate duties delegated to you. It is only fair that if we delegate to others, we must also be willing to accept an appropriate task that is delegated to us.

Avoiding Procrastination

Procrastination is defined as the chronic delay in implementing actions that accomplish important tasks. It is inaccurate to assume that procrastination is either good or bad. There may be times when delaying a task does not have adverse consequences. In other situations, consistently putting things off and not getting responsibilities completed could be very detrimental to accomplishing goals.

Davidson states that procrastination behavior begins in childhood. If a child is allowed to put things off, this often continues into adulthood (1978, p. 75). Studies show that only about 50 percent of people admit to being chronic procrastinators. Perhaps this reticence has to do with the fact that procrastinators in our society are looked upon as being lazy or disorganized. Some investigators think that procrastinators are basically insecure, easily distracted, perfectionistic, and possessed of a distorted time/future sense. This means that they cannot accurately predict how long a task will take.

People may procrastinate for several reasons. Procrastination can place responsibility on others rather than on oneself. Not doing the task may be rebellion against "those who are making me do something." Anxiety may be decreased because the task at hand can be put off, reducing the pressure. Some persons experience increased self-esteem or status because they have found the power necessary to delay a project if they choose.

Others who are fearful of failing at a task may put it off in the hope that it will just go away.

It is unfortunate when nurses procrastinate in areas related to patient care. Other staff members and supervisors may view the procrastinator nurse as undependable. Although clinically sound in providing the essentials of care, the nurse who procrastinates may give the appearance of being incompetent. The trust relationship between the nurse and the patient may be severed because of what the nurse considers to be an unimportant request.

Research in this area has been very limited, but it may be consoling to know that most of us procrastinate at one time or another. When procrastination becomes a habit leading to feelings of guilt and the perception on the part of others that we are unreliable, steps to change are clearly indicated.

Many techniques can help chronic procrastinators if they recognize that the behavior is a problem. Lakein states that "delay makes the task seem larger when you do get around to it" (1973, p. 135). Knowing this, tasks can be made more manageable if they are broken into pieces and done one part at a time. A project does not seem so overwhelming using this technique. Procrastinators should neither ask for nor be given more time on a project. This only intensifies the tendency to put off deadlines. Studying the principles of time management is very helpful. Procrastinators should also allow more time than they think a task will take. Another important step is to make a personal commitment for completion of a task by a deadline. For example, if you have a college assignment for Monday and would like to spend the weekend with your family, make a commitment that the assignment will be completed by 9 on Friday evening. Then, when you have completed a task in the time projected, give yourself a reward. In the situation just described, the reward is obvious: a special time with your family. At other times, you might buy yourself a special food item or a rose at the grocery store. These are tangible reminders that you have overcome the tendency to delay what needed to be done.

Reading Efficiently

Students have a great deal of assigned and professional reading. As a nurse, you will find that you must read widely to stay current. One of the best solutions is to take a course in speed reading. However, this may be impossible at the present time. There are, nevertheless, some techniques you can do. Focus first on the opening paragraph, the headings, the summary paragraph, and any charts or lists in a chapter. This gives you an overview of the contents and allows you to read more quickly through the remainder of the material. Underline important passages for study later. Between readings place texts and materials in a designated location so that you do not have to spend time looking for what you want.

Making Meetings More Productive

Many meetings waste time. You will be attending meetings of organizations to which you belong as well as nursing meetings and meetings of the health care team. An agenda should be prepared and circulated prior to a meeting, so that those attending know what is to be discussed ahead of time. This practice greatly decreases the time spent in lengthy discussions during the meeting. The most productive meetings last approximately 1 to 1.5 hours. After this period of time, effective decision making declines substantially because of participant distraction and fatigue. Meetings should convene and adjourn on time. Time is wasted when members who arrive on time have to wait for latecomers to arrive in order to begin. When adjournment is delayed and the meeting continues for an undetermined period of time, some members may need to leave. This diminishes the strength of the group. It has been suggested that meetings should be held with members standing; no chairs. Although this suggestion may not be taken seriously, meetings held in warm rooms with padded, comfortable chairs tend to be prolonged, because of the comfort and lack of attention of the members.

The use of ad hoc committees can greatly save time. An ad hoc committee is a designated smaller group of people who are assigned a specific task. The ad hoc committee reports back to the larger group after collecting information and/or making recommendations regarding the specific topic.

Planning Leisure

When we discussed making a "to do" list, we mentioned the importance of including leisure time. This is not wasted time. Leisure time regenerates our energy so that we can get more work done when we return to work. People commonly report feeling much better about doing tasks after cycling, walking, listening to music, or reading for pleasure. It has been suggested that leisure activities bring about a distinct change in brain metabolism that enhances task performance.

When working in the care setting, take breaks and meals as scheduled. Nurses who skip their time off the unit because they are "too busy" delude themselves. They become less efficient and overly fatigued without relief time.

Living a Healthy Life-style

Eating well maximizes the energy that we can direct toward employing time management techniques. During times of intense concentration on tasks, it is best to eat lightly but nutritiously. An August 1982, survey conducted by the National Restaurant Association found that the primary reasons persons in our society eat out is lack of time and for convenience. Most patronize fast food restaurants. You need not eat out to save time. You can listen to tapes while a salad or simple meal is prepared or meal preparation can become a time that can be shared with children, others in the family, or friends. The time when meals are eaten, however, should be one of leisure and enjoyment. Remember that heavy meals and alcoholic intake all decrease productivity.

Obtaining adequate rest and sleep also maximizes our energy. The quantity of rest and sleep needed is unique to each individual, and what is adequate for one person may not be adequate for another. It is well known that fatigue diminishes effectiveness on timed tasks.

Taping the Intershift Report

Taping the intershift report is another time saver in hospitals. Taping has many advantages, such as eliminating social and unrelated comments from listeners. It can be done at a convenient time near the end of a shift. The nurses who have taped the report can remain on the unit to meet patient needs while others listen to the report. The next shift of nurses has a taped record of the report that can be reviewed for points that need clarification. A disadvantage is the inability to clarify information while listening to the tape. It also takes skill on the part of the reporting nurse. At first, making notes ahead of time can be useful for the beginning nurse. However, proficiency can be easily achieved with practice.

Using Computers to Save Time

A growing number of homes have a computer. The prediction is that these will be used in the future for a variety of tasks, such as letter writing, balancing a check book, and shopping. Computers in health care are also time-saving devices. Their use ranges from the accessing of laboratory data to the formulation of nursing care plans and actual charting. Knowledge of the basics of a home computer can be transferred to use of the computer in the health care setting. In some health care settings computer literacy is a requirement. In others it is of growing interest for its efficiency and time-saving qualities. Many resources are available in the community to help the beginner learn these skills.

Two activities may help you in applying some of the time management principles we have discussed in this chapter. The first display is a list of time management techniques. Try implementing each one and evaluate its effectiveness for you. The second display is an exercise that provides you with a hypothetical situation. Making use of time management techniques, plan care for the five patients assigned to you on one shift as described on the form.

Time Management Techniques

- Write down your ideas; do not trust your memory.
- Have a single accessible calendar.
- Develop and consult a tickler file regularly.
- Make at "to do" list at home and in the clinical setting; set priorities and plans for delegating either early in the morning or at the end of the day.
- Structure in time for leisure.
- Concentrate on one project at a time.
- Appropriately bunch some items, such as errands.
- Carry 3 × 5 cards with you to jot down ideas.
- Carry reading material with you at all times for periods when you have to wait.
- Say no to time-consuming requests for which you do not have time.
- Use your high-energy hours for A projects and your low-energy hours for C's and easier projects.
- Find a place where you will not be interrupted.
- Only handle paper once.
- Have a place for everything.
- Shop in a familiar supermarket.
- Eat easy-to-fix but nutritious food and plan adequate exercise, rest, and sleep.
- Limit socializing in general.
- Limit unnecessary phone calls; perhaps use a home answering device.
- Use tapes during car travel.
- Identify tasks that can be delegated and choose willing, capable people.
- Be willing to accept delegation.
- Set reasonable deadlines for yourself and others.
- Work on big tasks in steps.
- Do not ask for extra time on projects; make a commitment.
- Underline important passages when reading.
- Work with a partner.
- Use an agenda when holding a meeting.
- Plan meetings to last not more than 1.5 hours.
- Use ad hoc committees when appropriate.

Applying Time Management Techniques to Nursing Practice

You are a staff nurse and arrive for report at 6:45. You find the following:

Short staff
Five patients
1. Prostatectomy patient, 2 days post-op
2. Cholecystectomy patient, 3 days post-op
3. Newly diagnosed cancer patient, colectomy; bleeding, coming back to the unit from ICU
4. Post-op "lap" patient coming back in 1 hour from surgery
5. Confused 85-year-old experiencing renal failure

Make a "to do" list.

Establish priorities.

Determine duties to be delegated.

SUMMARY

Learning to control time rather than have time control you can be a challenge and may be one of the most important things you can do for yourself. Having time to be more reflective and thoughtful is a blessing in a society caught up in the crunch of time. Is the stress imposed by time constraints contagious?

Increasing your time management skills can provide better control over your life, allow you to accomplish more in less time, decrease anxiety, increase satisfaction, and provide more leisure time. You will find that time management skills help you in both your personal and your professional life.

To learn to manage your time effectively you must first set goals. After you have determined your goals, you will need to assess your current time management. As you plan for changing your approach to time management you may want to try the suggestions offered for calendars, tickler files, "to do" lists, and setting priorities. The aids to time management offered are all techniques you can use to facilitate your own ability to manage time effectively. Of far-reaching importance is the question of whether we are passing on to our children the concept that "faster is better." Rushing from one activity to another gives this message. Prophetically, Gibbs states, "But at some point, individuals must find the time to consider the price of their preoccupation and the toll of the spirit exacted by exhaustion. With too little sleep there are too few dreams. And for children especially, being eight years old should include some long, ice-creamy afternoons of favorite stories and grassy feet. Some things are just worth the time" (1989, p. 67).

Study Questions/Activities

1. Describe how Western society views individuals and time.
2. How does time management affect personal and organizational economics?
3. Name three benefits of managing time effectively.
4. Give one example each of your personal and professional short-term and long-term goals.
5. Discuss the advantages of performing a time assessment exercise.
6. What are the differences between a calendar and a tickler file?
7. When setting priorities after making a "to do" list, how do you prioritize your B items?
8. Name five aids to time management and how you intend to incorporate them into your time management plan.
9. Using the five aids you named in question 8, describe how you intend to apply them to your personal life and your work as a nurse.
10. List the four basic guidelines to delegation.
11. Discuss several techniques for helping people who chronically procrastinate.
12. What time savers can be used that make meetings more productive?
13. How does living a healthy life-style relate to time management?
14. Briefly discuss taping intershift report and the use of computers as time-saving techniques relating to nursing.

REFERENCES

Davidson, J. (1978). *Effective time management: A practical workbook*. New York: Human Science Press.

Gibbs, N. (1989). How America has run out of time. *Time*. April 24, 65–67.

Lakein, A. (1973). *How to get control of your time and your life*. New York: New American Library.

Murphy, E.C. (1984). Delegation—From denial to acceptance. *Nursing Management.* 15(1), 54–56.

Rifkin, J. (1987). *Time wars: The primary conflict in human history*. New York: Henry Holt.

Webber, R.A. (1980). *Time is money: The key to managerial success*. New York: The Free Press.

SUGGESTIONS FOR FURTHER READING

Barkas, J.L. (1984). *Creative time management*. Englewood Cliffs, N.J.: Prentice-Hall.

Drucker, P.F. (1966). *The effective executive*. New York: Harper & Row.

Dorney, R.C.(1988). Making time to manage. *Harvard Business Review.* 60(1), 38–40.

Douglas, L.M. (1988). *The effective nurse manager*. St. Louis: C.V. Mosby.

Haber, P.C. (1982, May 3). Why some people are always late. *U.S. News and World Report,* pp. 49–50.

Haynes, M.E. (1985). *Practical time management*. Tulsa: PennWell Books.

Kron, T., & Gray, A. (1987). *The management of patient care*. Philadelphia: W.B. Saunders.

McAlvanak, M.F. (1988). Time management: A key to fulfilling job expectations. *Pediatric Nurse, 14*(6), 536.

Morris, S., & Charney, N. (1983, October). Whipping procrastination—Now. *Psychology Today,* pp. 80–81.

Predd, C.S. (1989). Great tips for setting priorities. *Nursing '89. 19*(10), 120–126.

Motivating Yourself and Others

8

Objectives

After completing this chapter, you should be able to:

1. *Define the terms* motive, motivator, *and* motivation.
2. *Explain why an understanding of motivation will enhance your nursing career.*
3. *Compare and contrast four popularly held theories of motivation and discuss their implications for the practice of nursing.*
4. *Explain how recent changes in society have had an impact on current human motivation.*
5. *Identify the key concepts of self-motivation and the factors affecting its development and its utilization.*
6. *Identify the key principles in successfully motivating others and the techniques you will need to be successful in this area.*
7. *Apply the strategies suggested in this chapter to your clinical practice.*

In any discussion about motives and motivation it is important to remember that people have many complex needs, all of which continually compete to drive their behaviors. No one person has exactly the same needs or intensity of needs as another.

The individual's needs, drives, and desires are his or her motives or intrinsic motivators. Extrinsic motivators are those factors outside the person—including money, work environment, and recognition—that drive the person. Motives are directed toward goals, which may or may not be conscious. Motives arouse and maintain activity and determine the general direction of an individual's behavior. Goals or incentives are the anticipated rewards toward which motives are directed. Motives are the reasons underlying behavior.

People differ not only in their *abilities* but in their *desires*. The strength of their desires constitutes their motivation. According to Mali (1978, p. 247) "motivation is motive strength, the intensity of the will to do, to meet or satisfy a need." The sequence for the development of the will to do is the following: (1) a want emerges; (2) wants become needs; (3) needs become motives; (4) motives become purposes to act; and (5) purposes to act become the will to do.

In this chapter you will be introduced to the research of four of the most respected contemporary social psychologists to help you to understand what factors motivate people. You will also learn what factors influence your motivation and how to make these factors work in your favor. Through a discussion of recent changes in society you will be able to see how these changes are affecting people's views of work. This will provide the background to the discussion of how to motivate others.

THEORIES OF MOTIVATION

Psychologists are interested in the motives of people because motives are the basis for behavior. They are interested in how these motives evolve from wants and needs and how those wants and needs drive people to develop and work toward goal achievement. According to motivational theorists, these wants and needs really cause behavior.

The principal objective of any theory on motivation is to explain the voluntary choices people make among a variety of possible behaviors. An introduction to the research and basic concepts of the best-known contemporary theorists will aid you in thinking analytically in specific situations. It is often important for you to understand what factors influence your motivation and the motivation of those around you in your work setting.

Abraham Maslow: Hierarchy of Needs

Perhaps the best-known and most frequently quoted contemporary theorist concerned with the hierarchy of needs is Abraham Maslow, a psychologist who developed his theory from research observations in an industrial setting (Maslow, 1954). Many present-day nursing program philosophies define humans as possessing a hierarchy of needs. The program you attend might be one of these.

According to Maslow, human needs are ordered in a hierarchy from simple to complex. The simplest needs, physiological needs, are the greatest behavior motivators until they are somewhat satisfied. Physiological needs are focused on survival—food, clothing, shelter. Until satisfied to the degree needed for sustaining life, most of a person's activities will be focused at this level. Other levels will provide no motivation. Once physiological needs have been gratified, security or safety needs become predominant—the need to feel protected, safe, free of fear. This is frequently referred to as the need for self-preservation. Once these two lower-level needs are fairly well satisfied, affiliation or acceptance will emerge as dominant. This is the need to be loved, to belong, and to be accepted by various groups. When affiliation needs become dominant, a person will strive for meaningful social relationships. Next, the person experiences the need for esteem, both self-esteem and recognition from others. Satisfaction of these esteem needs produces such feelings as self-confidence, prestige, power, and control. The final need on this hierarchy is the need for self-actualization—the need to maximize one's potential—"the desire to become more and more of what one is, to become everything that one is capable of becoming" (Maslow, 1954, p. 92).

In reality, most people in our society tend to be partially satisfied and partially dissatisfied on many different levels all at the same time. Usually, lower-level needs are more easily met than higher-level needs, however, and do not tend to dominate.

A person's dominant need level dictates his or her motivation. For example, money is an excellent motivator for people who are focused on physical needs, such as food and shelter. According to Maslow, prepotent motives are those that are being least satisfied and therefore are currently more prominent than others. Satisfied needs decrease in strength and normally do not motivate individuals to seek goals or incentives to continue to satisfy them.

Exclusive of such groups as the homeless and the urban poor, a large segment of our society does not have to worry about being hungry, without shelter, or unsafe. The American worker on whom this chapter will focus, has for the most part satisfied physiological and safety needs. This has been the result of a tremendous increase in our standard of living, minimum wage, fringe benefits, government subsidies, unions, and labor laws. Our society has an almost built-in guarantee of fulfillment of physiological and safety needs for a large segment of the population.

Maslow found in his industrial research studies that the work force of today is motivated by a desire for the fulfillment of higher-level needs both in and out of the work environment.

Frederick Herzberg: Motivation–Hygiene Theory

Herzberg (1959, 1966), while taking into account the research and theory development of Maslow, has approached needs and motivators from a different perspective. The development of his motivation–hygiene theory resulted from the analysis of data derived from a study that involved extensive interviews with over 200 engineers and accountants from industries in the Pittsburgh area. In these interviews, subjects were asked what factors in their jobs made them unhappy or dissatisfied and what factors made them happy or satisfied.

Herzberg concluded that humans have two different categories of needs that are essentially independent of each other and affect behavior in different ways. He found that when people felt dissatisfied with their jobs, they focused on the environment in which they were working. Conversely, when people felt satisfied with their jobs, they focused on work itself. Herzberg called the first category of needs dissatisfiers, or hygiene factors, because they described our environment and served the primary function of preventing job dissatisfaction. He called the second category of needs motivators or satisfiers, because they seemed to be effective in motivating people to superior performance.

Variables such as organizational policies, work conditions, interpersonal relationships, salaries, status, and job security were referred to as hygiene factors. These are not an intrinsic part of a job but are related to the conditions under which a job is performed. Herzberg's "hygienes" can be said to parallel Maslow's lower-level needs. The researcher relates his use of the word *hygienes* to its medical meaning—preventive and environmental. Hygiene factors, Herzberg says, do not induce people to make an extra effort; they only prevent losses in worker performance due to work restrictions.

Satisfying factors that involve feelings regarding the work itself— achievement, professional growth, recognition, responsibility, and advancement, which expand job challenge and scope—are referred to as *motivators*. Herzberg uses this term because these factors seem capable of having a positive effect on job satisfaction, often resulting in an increase in one's job efforts and output. Herzberg's motivators then can be said to parallel Maslow's level 4 and level 5 needs: esteem and self-actualization.

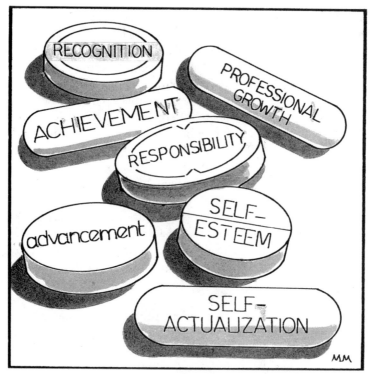

Satisfying factors that involve feelings about the work itself and that expand job challenge and scope are referred to as *motivators*.

Thus, hygiene needs, when satisfied, tend to eliminate dissatisfaction and work restriction but do little to motivate an individual to superior performance or increased capacity. Satisfaction of the motivators, however, permits an individual to grow in his or her job performance and, in turn, increase his or her abilities. What is really needed in the work environment, according to Herzberg, is job enrichment, by which he means the deliberate upgrading of responsibilities, scope, and challenge in work.

David McClelland: Affiliation—Power—Achievement

David McClelland and associates (1953, 1961) at Harvard University have studied motivational phenomena. They identified three major motivators: affiliation, power, and achievement. They defined affiliation in the same way Maslow does. Power is a motivator for those who feel a need for control and authority (see Chap. 4 for a discussion of power). McClelland focused much of his writing on the need for achievement and its importance in motivating many individuals. Through years of research and extensive data collection McClelland has been able to describe achievement-motivated people as possessing a desire to be successful in competitive situations. Achievement-motivated people set moderately difficult but potentially attainable goals for themselves; they like to assume responsibility for problem solving rather than leave the outcome to chance; they believe that their efforts and abilities can positively influence the outcomes of moderately risky situations.

Another characteristic of achievement-motivated people is that they seem to be more concerned with personal achievement than with the rewards these achievements may bring. Although rewards are not rejected, they are not as important as the accomplishment itself. Rewards are valuable primarily as a measure of personal performance. They provide a means of assessing progress toward goal achievement and an opportunity to measure personal accomplishments against the accomplishments of others.

As a corollary to this, achievement-motivated people often prefer situations in which they receive concrete feedback on their performance. They tend to value task-related feedback, rather than social–attitudinal feedback, most. The latter is far more important to people who are focused on the need for affiliation, as was mentioned earlier. Thus, if McClelland's theory were to be placed in the context of Maslow's hierarchy of needs, achievement-motivated people would be placed high on the hierarchy. They would be seen as people who for the most part had achieved satisfaction in the areas of physical needs, self-preservation needs, and acceptance needs.

McClelland postulates that achievement-motivated people spend a lot of time thinking about doing things better and that this thinking in achievement terms precipitates positive behaviors. The classic example is that of college students who possess high achievement needs; they generally receive better grades than equally bright students with weaker achievement needs.

McClelland has also found that achievement-motivated people are more likely to be from families in which high demands are made for independence and performance at an early age. These demands are commensurate with the ability level of the child, however. Accomplishments are favorably and liberally rewarded and thus build independence and self-confidence. In their adult lives, these people often seek reasonable challenges to meet their needs for achievement.

McClelland's research has demonstrated that, given certain circumstances, achievement needs can be an important motivator. Good job performance, for example, becomes very important, resulting in high motivation to perform well. Achievement motivation does not usually operate when people are performing routine or boring tasks in which no competition is involved. When challenge and competition are involved, however, achievement motivation will stimulate good performance.

In summary, the research on achievement motivation suggests that such motivation is most likely to be present when moderately challenging tasks have to be performed and an even chance of success is perceived; when competition is present; when performance is perceived to depend on a valued skill; and when performance feedback is given.

Douglas McGregor: Theory X and Theory Y

Douglas McGregor (1966) believed that the traditional structure of the work environment, where control and decision making were carried out at the top of the management pyramid, was based on a theory about humans that he labeled as Theory X. Theory X postulates that most people would rather be directed than assume any responsibility for creative problem solving, find work distasteful and are motivated primarily by physical and security needs, must be managed through close supervision, seek rewards in money and fringe benefits, and are coerced into positive performance with threats of punishment.

Drawing on Maslow's theory of the hierarchy of needs, McGregor concluded that Theory X's assumptions about the nature of humans are generally inaccurate because most people have satisfied their physical and safety needs and are therefore motivationally dominated by the needs for affiliation, esteem, and self-actualization. Enter Theory Y.

Theory Y assumes that people are basically reliable and naturally enjoy work if conditions are favorable; can be self-directed, can be creative, and welcome opportunities to make contributions; and can be motivated by exposure to progressively less external control and progressively more self-control.

Thus, McGregor believes that broadening individual responsibility is beneficial to both workers and the organizations for which they work. Giving people the opportunity to grow and mature on the job helps them to satisfy more than just physiological and safety needs. It motivates them to seek higher-level needs, utilize more of their potential, be more productive on the job, and thus achieve more of the needs of the organization and of their own needs. This philosophy and the theory on which it is based are often operationalized in organizations focused on increasing worker productivity. The different theories of motivation are summarized in Table 8-1.

6

TABLE 8-1. THEORIES OF MOTIVATION

Theory	Description	Application
Maslow Hierarchy of needs	Physiological (food, clothes, shelter) ↓ Self-preservation (safety, protection) ↓ Affiliation/acceptance (love, belonging) ↓ Esteem (self-confidence, recognition) ↓ Self-actualization (maximum achievement, competence)	Managers who facilitate opportunities for employees to meet more than basic needs in the work setting will attract and retain more and better workers.
Herzburg Motivation–hygiene	Dissatisfiers/hygiene factors (prevent job dissatisfaction) Focus on work environment, work conditions *versus* Satisfiers/motivators (promote superior performance); focus on work achievement	Managers who provide employees with job enrichment opportunities will increase worker performance
McClelland Affiliation, power, achievement	Major motivators: affiliation (need to belong) Power (need to control) Achievement (need to succeed)	Managers who are aware of employees' unique needs for motivators and provide appropriate opportunities for needs, gratification will stimulate superior work performance.
McGregor Theory X Theory Y	*Theory X* Workers are basically dissatisfied and are motivated by money and fringe benefits. *versus* *Theory Y* Workers are basically satisfied and welcome opportunities to be self-directed and creative.	Managers who broaden employees' responsibility will enhance their job productivity

SELF-MOTIVATION

Know Yourself

Identifying and analyzing human needs, their interrelatedness, and their power as motivators will provide a foundation on which to build an understanding of personal needs, motivators, and motivation. This has broad application to how you are able to keep yourself motivated for peak performance and how you can be instrumental in motivating those around you to enhance their performance.

According to Shinn (1981, p. 11), self-motivation is composed of two parts: "The first is mental: you conceive in your mind where you want to go. The second part is physical: you take action to get there. Mind and action are equally important. . . . Self-motivation—thought and action—is the key to success."

Where do *you* want to go? Arriving at an answer to this question may take a little soul searching, but this is the most important first step to success. Remember the saying, "If you don't know where you're going, you'll probably end up somewhere else" (Campbell, 1974).

Your most important resource in life is yourself. How well you understand yourself will determine how well you are able to set and achieve your goals. Who are you? What are your strengths and your weaknesses? The answers to these questions may not be as difficult as they seem at first.

In your program in nursing you are frequently called upon to evaluate your performance against the goals and objectives of the program of study. After each clinical rotation, for example, you may be required to complete a self-evaluation similar to the evaluation of your performance that you receive from your instructor. On these evaluations you are encouraged to analyze your personal goals and to strive to make them realistically attainable yet congruent with the goals of the program in nursing. In these exercises you are encouraged to be reflective, objective, and honest.

These familiar and frequently repeated exercises have no doubt become increasingly more comfortable for you. In addition to heightening your self-awareness, they serve to prepare you for the real world of nursing.

By helping you to get to know yourself better, to understand your personal wants and needs (motives), and to capitalize on your strengths and minimize your weaknesses, you have grown in your ability to use this most valuable resource—yourself. The feedback you receive from your instructors helps you continually to reassess yourself in an increasingly more objective way. Most important, repeated self-evaluation helps you to incorporate information into appropriate and realistic goal setting for the future. When you are able to judge yourself objectively, you can make the right first step to job satisfaction through goal setting.

Set Goals

The difference between achieving and not achieving lies in setting goals. Having and using a goal-achievement action plan will promote your career growth. The key purpose of setting goals is to find out what you want out of life. According to Calano and Salzman (1988), most people conduct their careers according to other people's expectations: "If you don't have the courage to pursue your own goals, you leave yourself open to the many people who will be only too happy to recruit you to pursue theirs!" (1988, p. 21).

If you wish to get ahead you can motivate yourself by identifying the goals you wish to reach, goals that you will work toward as you develop your talents. Therefore, you need a plan. Plans are to your personal life what blueprints are to the contractor building a house. You need this blueprint as your plan of action to aid you in developing your talents so that you can achieve your specific goals. Remember, these goals should be your goals, not those of someone else.

Develop an Action Plan

Following is a list of the steps that you will need to take to reach your goals.

Step 1. *Prioritize goals.* Your goals should be in writing. This will help you to prioritize them. Some goals are obviously more important than others. Prioritizing goals will help you focus and direct your energies appropriately. An example of a goal related to your clinical performance might be to become a successful, effective team leader.

Step 2. *List steps to achievement.* You should list steps to achievement. This is your action plan. It should be realistic and time limited. Identify objectives or short-term intermediate steps. This will make the accomplishment of long-range goals easier because it will prevent you from feeling overwhelmed and will provide you with a psychological lift when the short-term intermediate steps have been reached. Using the example of becoming a successful team leader again, one of your objectives might be to read four journal articles on effective team leading that you found in your suggested reading list. You might set reading one article each night for the next four nights as your objective.

Step 3. *Identify positive qualities.* Listing your positive qualities will help achieve your objectives. This will help you feel optimistic about your ability to achieve your goals. For example, you may have developed good communication skills or you may work well with people.

Step 4. *List deficiencies.* List your deficiencies. You know you are a procrastinator, for example, and although your intentions are good, you often waste time avoiding what you know you need to do. This chapter will discuss overcoming such deficiencies.

Step 5. *Weigh strengths and weaknesses.* Weighing strengths and weaknesses will help you to be more realistic about what you can accomplish and will help you to avoid setting your goals so high that they are never achievable and that you are therefore constantly frustrated. This action will also help you to face up to your weaknesses and develop the contingency plan necessary to overcome them.

Step 6. *Review plan.* Reviewing your action plan frequently will help you assess your progress, face up to obstacles encountered along the way, identify alternate courses of action if necessary, and redefine your goals. This will move you toward goal attainment.

When developing your list of goals, it is important to keep specific goal characteristics in mind. The goals you identify for yourself should be

- Written and prioritized
- Clear and specific
- Action oriented and measurable
- Realistic and compatible
- Flexible
- Time limited
- Both short and long range.

Increase Self-Esteem

According to Charles Garfield, author of *Peak Performance* (1984), the ability to succeed is something you learn, not something with which you are born. What keeps you from achieving your potential, your "peak performance," is first and foremost not believing in yourself, not believing that you can do it!

Developing the kinds of habits and skills that will lead you to goal achievement depends in large part on your self-esteem. The higher your self-esteem, the more easily you will face up to and conquer your weaknesses, your high stress level, and your frequent procrastination. The better you are able to face up to and conquer your weaknesses, the higher your self-esteem will rise. It is a circular and self-perpetuating process that, when adopted, can positively change your life.

When your self-esteem is high you solve problems by focusing on a solution, not by placing blame on someone else. When your self-esteem is high you get involved and take reasonable risks rather than leaving life's situations to chance. When your self-esteem is high you view failure as an opportunity to learn and grow and you try again—and again—and again, until you succeed. Best of all, when your self-esteem is high you feel better about yourself, you project a more positive image, and those around you begin to feel better about you in turn.

There is probably little doubt that you agree with what has been said so far about the merits of positive self-esteem. The problem is knowing how to develop and improve your self-esteem.

Look and Act Your Best

Although it is not the purpose of this chapter to expound on the type of life-style habits that promote good mental and physical health, or to discuss diet and exercise, or rest and diversion, it is important to reinforce briefly how these factors affect the image you project.

How you look affects how you feel about yourself. If you feel you look your best, you have more self-confidence. An attractive appearance is also a statement to the rest of the world. If you are not motivated enough to respect yourself, you cannot expect to motivate others to respect you either.

How you act is as important as how you look. You must project yourself so that others respond to you in the way you want. Ask yourself, "What are some of the qualities that I admire in others that I should strive to develop in myself?" Give this some serious thought.

Use Affirmations and Visualizations

Do you have a little voice in your head that is constantly putting you down with comments such as "I'm too fat," "I'd lose my head if it wasn't attached," or "I never was the brainy type"? This voice needs to be reprogrammed to help you build your self-esteem and create a successful pattern. This reprogramming occurs when you turn these negative statements into positive statements: "I look great just the way I am;" "I'm responsible and reliable;" "I am as capable of achieving as anyone else." These positive statements are called affirmations. Affirmations help you to increase your self-esteem, project a more confident self-image, and help others to see you in a better light.

A similar technique is called *visualization*. Instead of using words, you use pictures to increase your self-esteem. In other words, you see yourself or visualize yourself as thin, as reliable, as confident. Soon you begin to adopt the behaviors that fit the image. Dressing the part and acting the part are the keys to success with this strategy.

Find a Role Model or Mentor

Find a role model or mentor. A role model is someone you would like to emulate. Observing this person in action will help you identify the specific behaviors you need to develop to reach your goal. A mentor is someone who has taken an interest in your development and who will help you work toward achieving your goals. If you make it your goal to surround yourself with positive people, people who look at a glass of water and see it as half full rather than as half empty, you will find the role models and mentors that will motivate you toward the positive actions you will need to take to increase your self-image.

Develop Your Talents

You have a number of talents. Some you are aware of; some are yet to be discovered and developed. It is your responsibility to continue to nurture your identified talents and to uncover and put to work your hidden talents.

Be Enthusiastic

You can develop and nurture your enthusiasm. Enthusiasm is a mixture of curiosity, confidence, expectation, and optimism. It is a positive self-expectancy of winning. Do not forget that the big difference between a winner and a loser is that a winner expects to win whereas a loser expects to lose. The degree of your motivation is in direct proportion to the amount of enthusiasm you possess.

Enthusiasm is not just positive thinking; it also incorporates the actions that support that positive thinking. Enthusiasm is the fuel that fires up your positive thinking and helps you turn this thinking into action.

The nice thing about enthusiasm is that it tends to help you rid yourself of stress. It is impossible to entertain these two emotions at the same time. When you are able to lower your stress level, you can change problems into challenges, focus on solutions, and resolve issues in your life much more quickly.

Another nice thing about enthusiasm is that it is contagious. Your enthusiasm will motivate and inspire others. It causes others to view you as the type of person they prefer to be around.

Enthusiasm helps you believe in yourself and your goals. It helps you believe that if your goals are realistic, they can be achieved. When you can harness your enthusiasm into action, you have put to use one of life's best motivators.

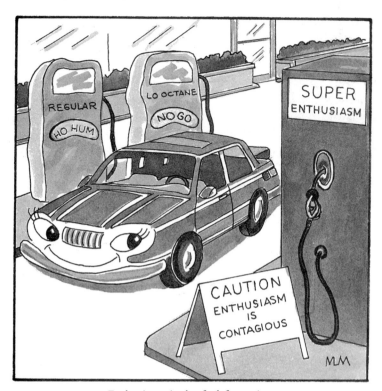

Enthusiasm is the fuel for action.

Be Creative

Creativity, like enthusiasm, is a talent that can be cultivated and released to become a powerful tool in motivating you to reach your goals. Constantly releasing your mental powers through creativity can become a habit. You will discover that answers and solutions will begin to come to you more quickly and with the expenditure of less energy.

One of the best ways to cultivate and nurture your creativity is to expose yourself continually to new ideas. Read your professional journals. They are a reliable source of state-of-the-art practices and research. Become more involved in the world around you. You learn so much more by being a participant rather than just an observer. Listen, and listen actively. Remember, you never learn anything new by talking, only by listening. Align yourself with creative people. Engage them in stimulating exchanges, such as brainstorming, to help you trigger your mind to release new ideas. As with most things in life, the more you engage in the activity, the more natural it becomes.

Be Flexible

One of life's few constants is change. Change permeates every aspect of our lives. If you are afraid of or resistant to it, you will not grow. What is even worse, you will inhibit the growth of those with whom you deal most regularly. How you react to and handle change and even how much you are willing to be a change agent will determine whether you succeed and move ahead or are left behind. Growth means having the courage and confidence to explore new options and as a result to let go of comfortable but outdated ones. Growth involves a certain amount of risk taking that can be both frightening and sometimes even painful, but success is the outcome that you can legitimately expect to attain.

Take Action

A mature approach to working toward independence is to take an increasing amount of responsibility. Do not always wait to be told what to do. Ask questions, volunteer to help others, get involved. The difference between minimally meeting objectives and excelling is taking charge of your own learning. Consider the description of the entry-level nurse as the base of your practice, not the boundary. Some of your best opportunities for initiative lie in the aspects of your job that nobody wants. Volunteer. Because nobody wanted the job in the first place, it is doubtful that anyone will bother to help you do it. Here is your chance for a little independence. At the very least your efforts will be appreciated, but more than likely the rewards will be far greater than that.

It is not what you know but what you do with what you know that counts. You should not be afraid to act, even though some risk is involved. Recognize that action is a learning process. An important part of action is the willingness to work hard. Give your very best in devotion and dedication to your project. If you wait for the assurance that everything will turn out perfectly, you will never act.

Action can be a therapy because it tends to erase doubts and fears. Even if you give 100 percent and for some reason fall short of your goal, there is tremendous satisfaction in knowing that you worked to the best of your ability to achieve. You certainly will have learned a great deal from the process and be richer for the experience.

MOTIVATING OTHERS

Now that you have a better understanding of what motivation is and how to get and keep yourself motivated, you are being asked to build on and apply this information to a discussion of how to motivate others. In your role as a beginning nurse it will definitely be part of your job to motivate your subordinates—the LPNs and nurse assistants whose care you direct. You might even be able to apply some of the information gained in this section to motivating your peers. That would make your job easier and more pleasant. You might even be able to motivate your immediate superiors by the examples you set. That would go a long way toward keeping you motivated.

Much of your success as a team leader or charge nurse directing or delegating to staff less qualified than you will depend on your people management skills—your ability to motivate those around you. In the final analysis, you will be judged not only on your own performance but on the performance of your team. The key to success in this area is to develop the kinds of relationships with your peers and subordinates that positively affect their behavior and work performance. At times this may even include getting them to do and feel as you do. The skill is in getting your team either to be happy to follow you or to be unaware that they are being led. The most successful motivators often become the most successful leaders. They are the people who cause things to happen. They move others to action with their ability to influence.

A Changing Society

Current conditions in society are changing the way people think about work. It is important to any discussion of motivating people, therefore, to review briefly these trends and how they impact on your ability to succeed in this area.

Attitudes Toward Authority

The line between labor and management is becoming more and more blurred. There has been a steady decline over the past couple of decades in the public's respect for institutional power and authority. There also has been a steady decline in traditional values and the traditional way of doing things. Today's workers are better educated, less responsive to authority figures, and usually quick to question a directive rather than just carrying it out. The collective strength of workers who are unionized adds still another dimension to the changing attitudes toward authority figures. This situation has the positive effect of forcing managers to involve workers in the decision-making process. In some situations, however, unionization has promoted mediocrity, because rewards are given across the board and there is little incentive for superior performance.

Work Ethic

Work is no longer central to people's lives. Years ago young workers were satisfied with a regular paycheck and a roof over their heads. This attitude toward work has been replaced by an attraction for the "good life," with all the emphasis on pleasure and leisure that this implies. This attitude has now permeated the workplace itself. Workers expect to experience quality in their work lives as well as in their private lives. This is directly related to the growing affluence of a large segment of our society. There is a de-emphasis on the necessities of life and an emphasis on seeking gratification of a higher-level need, that of self-fulfillment.

Their social commitment is also becoming increasingly important for many people. They are becoming more and more aware of the need to be connected with their community, of how their work affects their community, and of how their work gives them an identity within their community. When work loses its value to employees, it becomes increasingly difficult to motivate them to perform at their best level or sometimes even to come to work at all!

Participation

Today's workers are more educated, more informed, more independent, more aware, more secure, more affluent than their predecessors. When they are performing tasks about which they know as much or more than their superiors, they expect to be consulted about those tasks, to have their input sought, to be listened to, to be respected for their knowledge and skills.

Mobility

We are a much more mobile society. Not only is travel made easier by the conveniences of modern transportation such as the airline shuttles that provide hourly service between many major cities, but also workers attitudes toward travel have changed. It is not uncommon to find people who travel to work each day for long distances over superhighways, who keep efficiency apartments close to work for use during the week and who go home on the weekends, or who work out of their homes. Such mobility and flexibility have broadened workers' job options and made it less important for them to feel committed to a single job or even a single area.

Nursing Shortage

The demand for nurses and nurse assistants is greater than the supply. This increases an employee's confidence level about obtaining and retaining a job. In some situations this could be a demotivator to job performance. Some might think, "They're desperate; they'll have to put up with my being late. It's better than not coming to work at all!"

Factors in Motivating Others

All the previously mentioned trends in our society will have an influence in your ability to motivate others. Simply put, you will need to be more aware, more sensitive, and more committed to your goal in order to be successful. Following is a discussion of the key factors you will need to consider in meeting your objective of motivating others.

Establish Credibility

You must establish yourself as someone whom your subordinates can trust and believe in. This trust becomes firmly established when you consistently follow up on all requests and problems and when you keep all promises. Trust in your judgment and ability to lead results when you are knowledgeable about patient care, rules and procedures, and all things that make you a valuable resource to your subordinates. Thus, you should strive to be respected for both your knowledge and your integrity.

The way you organize your time (see Chap. 7) and balance it against your priorities should provide a model for those you want to motivate. If you are floundering, you are not much of an inspiration to someone else. Projecting that you are unsure of yourself and your direction will cause the people who depend on you to feel the same. As Buck Rogers states in his book *Getting the Best Out of Yourself and Others* (1987, p. 29), "Once you're in a management position you're a role model, like it or not. You set the tone and the pace. You control the energy level. You define the ethics. You impart to your people the importance and seriousness of what they and you do."

You do not always have to be in a leadership position to be a role model and motivate others, however, as the following example demonstrates. A nurse tells the story of her colleague with whom she had the pleasure of working. They were employed on a busy medical–surgical floor. This colleague was determined that all her clients were going to have written Kardex care plans. She was also determined that this would not mean that the task would be drudgery or that she would have to stay long after her scheduled work hours to meet her objective.

Her drive to and from work was about 20 minutes each way, 30 minutes if she met heavy traffic. She had a tape recorder in her car and began to use her travel time to dictate her thoughts about the nursing care needs of one of her clients on her way to work and about those of another client on her way home. If she ran into traffic, she could often focus on the needs of two clients.

When she got to work, she would play back the tape and transcribe her thoughts into the Kardex during her break. She never pushed others to follow her example, but it soon became apparent to her coworkers that this plan was very effective and time-saving. Her colleagues liked to care for her clients on her days off too, because the updated care plans helped them prioritize care.

Soon others began to adopt the same plan. An informal contest developed among the group to see if every client on the unit could have a care plan. A little peer pressure also developed, which served to keep the momentum going. The unit secretary even got motivated to become involved and would transcribe the taped care plans into the Kardex when time permitted. For the most part, this unit continues to boast of written Kardex care plans for 100 percent of its clients.

Some of the fringe benefits of this activity have been a sense of common goals and purposes leading to a cohesive team effort, more knowledgeable and more time-efficient client care, and lack of frustration with the drive to work. There has been some road construction in the area of the hospital this past year, and the nurses on this unit are the only ones who arrive at work unruffled from the drive. They develop two care plans instead of one each morning!

Take an Interest in Others

One of the greatest motivators is caring. All human beings like to feel that someone cares about them. Remember what Maslow said about affiliation or acceptance—the need to be loved, to belong, to be accepted? If you are able to meet that need in your subordinates, they will be very motivated to return the favor by helping you achieve the goals of client care that you have set for your team.

What skills will you need to do this? The single most important behavior for you to exhibit is a genuine interest in the members of your staff as individuals. This focus should be on their job performance, not on their personal life, however. Take an interest in their careers and help them grow. This can be done by exposing them to new ideas and new ways to do things. When you see that people are ready for a little more responsibility, give it to them. When possible, include your nurse assistants in team discussions about patients. You might be pleasantly surprised at the suggestions they make. Include as many of your team as possible in inservice programs, even if they are not going to be directly responsible for the information or equipment discussed.

Take an interest in their upward mobility. Encourage them to go back to school and offer to help them by answering questions or rearranging their work schedules when possible.

The now famous Hawthorne Experiments (Mayo, 1945) proved, better than any words might, the power of caring. In 1927 a Harvard Business School professor, Elton Mayo, began to conduct a series of experiments at the Western Electric Company's Hawthorne plant in

Illinois. His original hypothesis was that better working conditions would improve productivity. Mayo began by improving lighting conditions. As he expected, productivity improved with better lighting. The interesting thing was, however, that in the control group, where the lighting conditions remained unchanged, productivity also went up. Unable to explain this, Mayo tried another experiment. In this experiment he divided the workers into three groups. For one group he improved the lighting conditions, in the second he left them the same, and in the third he made them worse. Much to his amazement, productivity improved in all three groups! In open-ended interviews that followed these experiments, Mayo found that workers expressed gratitude that someone was paying attention to them and making them feel important. Mayo's conclusion, often referred to as the "Hawthorne effect," was that what really caused the improvement in motivation and performance in these workers was the attention paid to them—the demonstration of caring.

Reward Positive Behaviors

"If high pay and generous benefit plans were enough to boost performance levels, the General Motors work force would be outperforming Toyota three to one" (Tarkenton, 1986. p. 20). Recall the earlier discussions in this chapter about the experiments done by Herzberg that led him to his motivation–hygiene theory? Out of all the factors that Herzberg identified as motivators, the two that ranked the highest were recognition and achievement. Some of your best motivators are related to the recognition you give your subordinates for a job well done.

You should develop the habit of recognizing extra effort and rewarding this behavior to reinforce it. A simple thank you is often enough. You may not be in a position to influence a subordinate's salary, although the writing of a fair and objective performance evaluation, discussed elsewhere in this book, might be one of your responsibilities.

Your genuine pleasure in a subordinate's extra efforts, your thoughtfulness in verbalizing it, and your effort to acknowledge it as close to its occurrence as possible are extremely powerful motivators. Unlike the performance evaluation, this is something you are assured of being able to control. Moreover, you should not keep good works secret. A public "thank you" carries much more power as a motivator than a private one. This might even motivate other team members to act in such a way as to receive the same reward. You should never miss a *legitimate* opportunity to add to an employee's pride and self-confidence. The word *legitimate* is emphasized for a reason. As with all motivational techniques, moderation, reasonableness, and, of course, sincerity are critical. Overzealous or insincere praise is as meaningless as no praise at all.

Fran Tarkenton (1986) has some interesting perspectives to share on

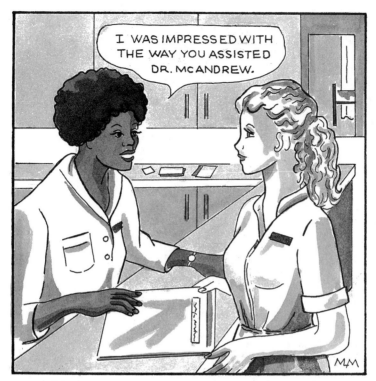

Some of the best motivators are related to recognition that you give to your subordinates for a job well done.

the topic of praise. He points out that most people you will be called upon to motivate will not be superstars, just ordinary, adequate workers. These will be the people that you will ignore, because you will probably make time to correct those that are doing a poor job and you will find it hard to ignore a true superstar. But what about the ordinary workers, who probably make up about 95 percent of the people you will be called upon to motivate? Tarkenton suggests that they should not be ignored. He explains his "4:1 Syndrome" (1986, p. 14):

> In most human situations,—given reasonably clear directions about what they're supposed to be doing, most people will do a good job about four times as frequently as they will do a below-par job . . . The person who works well four days out of five ought to be praised four times as often as he's dumped on. But, guess what? That's exactly the opposite of what happens . . . [a person] will work well 80 percent of the time, but 80 percent of the comments that his [superior] makes to him will focus on that 20 percent of the time he is performing under par. The 80 percent of the time he works well will simply go by without comment, because that's what he's "supposed" to be doing.

Many studies have shown that in the absence of positive feedback, performance will stay just above the level where a reprimand would likely occur. There is a tendency for the average worker to do just what he or she can safely get away with and no more, unless he or she is given a reason to increase his or her performance and is somehow motivated.

What other measures might you employ to reward your subordinates exclusive of praise? You could share your observations and appreciation with *your* superior. You could offer to include your subordinate in an inservice program. You could rearrange the schedule to accommodate one of his or her social events. You could take him or her to coffee. You could offer him the opportunity to take on a new assignment.

Consider these truisms when evaluating the significance of rewarding positive behaviors:

- Positive behaviors that are reinforced by praise tend to continue or even increase.
- Negative behaviors that are demotivated by withdrawing rewards tend to diminish.
- Positive behaviors that are not rewarded tend to diminish or even disappear over time.

Offer Constructive Criticism

Do not be fooled into believing that your success with motivating others can be achieved through friendship. It is important to have a pleasant, cordial working relationship that is grounded in mutual respect, but not in a close and personal friendship. Being the most popular member of the team is not being an effective motivator of others if your popularity stems from always giving in or compromising your standards in order to be liked. Rather, what *is* needed is the ability to get along with people in a way that strengthens and enhances your position.

At the opposite end of the spectrum are the use of scare tactics. Although scare tactics are motivational, they do far more to motivate your subordinate to look for another job than they do to motivate that person to do his or her present job well. This approach is usually adopted by someone who takes pleasure in destroying a subordinate's self-esteem. You've already seen how important self-esteem is to motivation. If you look closely, you will find that this approach is often adopted by someone with a very fragile ego who must constantly prove himself or herself. The damage done to the employee's pride and morale is inexcusable and unfortunately often difficult to repair. People who are approached in this manner are less productive and definitely less creative. So everyone loses!

This could be referred to as the *buddy to bully continuum*. You cannot effectively motivate by being a best friend or by being taken advantage of or by never setting standards just to maintain popularity. By the same token, you cannot expect to motivate anyone to come through for you in a tough situation, give that extra effort on a busy day, or share a truly creative idea if you treat everyone as unworthy.

What do you do? Like it or not, part of your motivational power is the leverage you have to discipline or control assignments and work environments. Rules and regulations are established to help things run smoothly and fairly. If they are not implemented and supported, they lose their meaning. Employees who abide by them are confused and demoralized when they see that those who do not follow these rules and regulations do so without consequence.

To put this into perspective, however, nobody should have to follow orders blindly that are not understood or that cannot be adequately explained to them. Further, no one should be punished for a first-time offense if it does not violate an established ethical, moral, or legal code or seriously jeopardize a client's physical or mental safety. Some people will feel the need to test you to see if you will back up your rules and live by your standards.

In this context the consequence should fit the error. Overreaction or unreasonable reprimands will often cause the subordinate to become afraid to make even the most minor decisions without constantly clearing them with you, which can be very time-consuming. An even worse scenario is that your subordinate becomes so anxious that he develops an error-prone behavior. Be reasonable. Be fair. Treat others the way you would want to be treated. Above all else, just as you praise in public, criticize in private!

Adapt the following perspective. If you do not offer constructive criticism to your subordinates, you rob them of their chance to improve. Not only is that thought important for you to keep in mind, but it might be worth sharing with the person you need to correct.

Here are some helpful hints for how to work with people who need constructive criticism:

- Be clear about your expectations and your directions to your subordinates.
- Give them suggestions as to how the improvement can be made.
- Give them reasonable opportunity to improve.
- Give the necessary reprimand and/or consequence at the time of the incident.
- Make the consequence appropriate to the error.
- Be consistent.
- Correct the behavior, not the person.
- Give credit for improvement when it occurs.

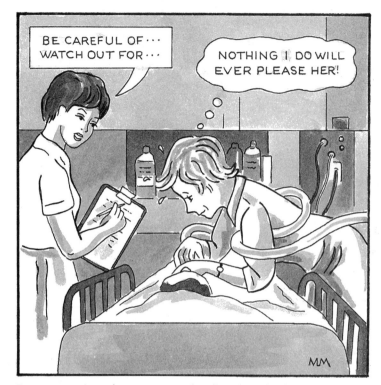

Frequent reprimands may cause subordinates to develop anxious and error-prone behavior.

Share Decision Making

People perform better when they feel they are contributing to a team effort, understand how their jobs fit into the overall scheme of things, and understand how their performance affects the team's performance. All people need to feel important. If team members do not think they make a difference and only think of their jobs as inconsequential and menial, they cannot experience job satisfaction or be high achievers. People work better when they can show off their talents, skills, and experiences.

There is a wonderful example shared by Hersey and Blanchard (1969, p. 50) that not only demonstrates the importance of involving subordinates in decision making but proves that this approach can work even with people who have low-level responsibilities.

A supervisor was transferred to a new plant. He was immediately confronted with a housekeeping problem. Complaints flooded into his office regarding how lazy and unmotivated the janitors were and how messy the work areas were. The supervisor immediately called a meeting of the janitors. He approached the group by acknowledging their expertise in the area of cleaning and asked them to help him solve the problem of the unsatisfactory work areas. With some encouragement from the supervisor the janitors became very verbal about the problems. Many of the problems stemmed from the janitors' feelings that they were not appreciated.

After that meeting the supervisor referred all housekeeping problems to the janitors. When salesmen came to the company to sell cleaning products, the supervisor referred them to the janitors. He gave the janitors the responsibility of making all decisions related to housekeeping, including the company from which to buy cleaning equipment. He gave the janitors an office for their personal use. As you might guess, almost overnight the company work areas became spotless. The janitors were made to feel important and in control. They took very seriously their responsibility of testing new products and dealing with salesmen. When you allow your subordinates to have this type of very basic control over their work, you demonstrate that you trust not only their judgment but also their loyalty.

The most challenging people to motivate are not usually those who do not have a lot of skill. You can often work with those individuals to develop necessary skills and help them to experience a sense of pride. You motivate them by using this approach. The problem is more often with people who may be overqualified for the job they have. How do you keep those persons interested and motivated? You do it by letting go—delegating appropriately. If you are going to be an effective motivator, you must understand that employees need to feel challenged but not threatened or intimidated.

What about situations in which you want to get your subordinates involved but are concerned about their ability to handle responsibility? This is where mutual goal setting and decision making become important. The key thing is to give your subordinate the opportunity to articulate his thoughts, opinions, and even the goals and objectives he has personally set for himself. This provides you with the opportunity to assess whether these goals and objectives are compatible with yours and those of the agency. If your subordinates ideas and goals are not compatible, you owe it to them to help bring them in line or to develop a mutually acceptable compromise. If they have no goals or have not thought them through, here is an opportunity for you to be helpful. Remember, as was illustrated earlier, goal setting is an important personal motivator. Keep in mind that just as your expectations must be articulated and understood by your subordinates, so must their expectations of you be allowed to be expressed. The more open the discussion, the less chance there will be for confusion when things are hectic and there is no time to establish ground rules.

Improve Communication Skills

Communication skills are directly tied to motivation, because if you hope to get anybody to do what you want, you must be able to communicate effectively. There are of course two components to communication: listening to what others are saying and telling others what you want. Many people feel that listening is even more important than speaking. Although it is true that we all have two ears but only one mouth, most people act as if the opposite were true. Over and over again research has born out that the average person only hears and understands about 25 percent of what is being said to him or her. This is in part due to the fact that people tend to listen in a passive way and do not get "involved" by focusing on the speaker and trying to integrate the message.

Some of the problems with understanding communications are that language itself can be very ambiguous. Not only do words themselves have several shades of meaning, but a person's background or experiences might cause him or her to interpret a message differently from its original intent. What is actually said and how the person looks and acts when he or she says it can be in direct conflict. This can result in a great deal of confusion for the person who is receiving the message. Aside from paying better attention, the best way to make sure that you understand what is being said to you is to clarify when in doubt. This is accomplished by "reflecting" back to the speaker what you perceived to be the message. You might say, "Now, if I understand you correctly, you are asking me. . . . " When it is your turn to send the message, make sure your message is clear, concise, and to the point. Summarizing or repeating a key point or two might be helpful. Remembering that receivers only integrate about 25 percent of what you are saying, you might want to ask them to use the same reflective technique on you that you used on them. See Chapter 10 for more information on communication.

SUMMARY

An individual's needs, drives, and desires are his or her motives or motivators. Motives are directed toward goals. Goals are the anticipated rewards toward which motives are directed. A person's motivation is his or her desire "to do." The motivation of an individual depends on the strength of his or her motives.

Many behavioral theorists have attempted to explain what motivates people to behave as they do. Four of the most widely accepted theories on motivation are presented in this chapter. Maslow's theory (hierarchy of needs) was developed around the idea that people have a group of needs that are arranged in a hierarchy from simple to complex and that simple needs, such as the need for food and shelter, must be satisfied before more complex needs, such as the need for self-esteem, can be addressed. Herzberg (motivation–hygiene theory) felt that people have two different and and distinct needs categories. The first category he called hygienes, which are mostly environmental in nature and serve to prevent dissatisfaction but do not motivate. The second category of needs he called motivators, because they affect people's motivation to increase their performance. McClelland (affiliation–power–achievement) concentrated his research on achievement as a motivator and described the characteristics of the achievement-motivated person. McGregor (Theory X and Theory Y) stated that according to Theory X, people are basically lazy, are motivated by rewards, and need to be coerced to produce. According to Theory Y, which McGregor supported, people are basically anxious to do a good job and are motivated by being recognized for a job well done and by being given more responsibility.

Your most important resource in life is yourself. How well you understand yourself will determine how well you are able to set and achieve your goals. If you wish to be successful, you can motivate yourself by identifying the goals you wish to reach, developing a plan of action, putting that plan to work, and reevaluating it frequently. By building and nurturing your self-esteem and identifying and putting your talents to work for you, you can develop the kind of habits and skills that will lead you to goal achievement.

To understand how to motivate others it is important to understand first how changes in values and changes in society affect people's motives. Changing attitudes toward authority and the work environment itself as well as the mobility of our population and the shortage of nurses have all had profound effects on worker motivation. Suggestions for incorporating ideas and concepts about motivating others into your everyday practice include establishing your credibility, taking an interest in others, rewarding positive behavior, offering constructive criticism, sharing decision making, and improving communication skills.

Study Questions/Activities

1. Define the terms *motives, motivators,* and *motivation.*
2. Explain why developing your self-motivation and being able to motivate others will enhance your nursing practice.
3. Compare and contrast the research of the four theorists introduced in this chapter and explain the value of their contributions to the understanding of motivation.
4. Give five examples of ways you could motivate yourself.
5. Give five examples of how you could motivate others.

6. Give a concrete example from your clinical experience of how and where information presented in this chapter could be put to use.

REFERENCES

Calano, J., & Salzman, J. (1988). *Career tracking.* New York: Simon & Schuster.
Campbell, D. (1974). *If you don't know where you're going, you'll probably end up somewhere else.* Allen, Texas: Argus Communications.
Garfield, C. (1984). *Peak performance.* New York: William Morrow.
Hersey, P., & Blanchard, K. (1969). *Management of organizational behavior.* Englewood Cliffs, N.J.: Prentice-Hall.
Herzberg, F., et al. (1959). *The motivation to work.* New York: John Wiley.
Herzberg, F. (1966). *Works and the nature of man.* New York: World Publishing Co.
Hill, N. (1983). *Think and grow rich.* New York: Fawcett Crest.
Mali, P. (1978). *Improving total productivity.* New York: John Wiley.
Maslow, A. (1954). *Motivation and personality.* New York: Harper & Row.
Mayo, E. (1945). *The social problems of an industrial civilization.* Cambridge, Mass.: Harvard University Press.
McClelland, D., et al. (1953). *The achievement motive.* Norwalk, Conn.: Appleton-Century-Crofts.
McClelland, D., et al. (1961). *The achieving society.* Princeton, N.J.: Van Nostrand.
McGregor, D. (1966). *Leadership and motivation.* Cambridge, Mass.: MIT Press.
Rogers, B. (1987). *Getting the best out of yourself and others.* New York: Harper & Row.
Shinn, G. (1981). *The miracle of motivation.* Wheaton, Ill.: Tyndale House.
Tarkenton, F. (1986). *How to motivate people.* New York: Harper & Row.

SUGGESTIONS FOR FURTHER READING

Arnold, J. (1978). *The art of decision-making.* New York: AMACOM.
Blake, R.R., & Mouton, J.S. (1981). *Productivity the human side.* New York: AMACOM.
Bliss, E.C. (1983). *Doing it now.* New York: Charles Scribner's Sons.
Burka, J., & Yuen, L. (1985). *Procrastination.* Reading, Mass.: Addison-Wesley.
Burns, D.D. (1980). *Feeling good: The new mood therapy.* New York: William Morrow.
Cherrington, D. (1980). *The work ethic.* New York: AMACOM.
Drucker, P.F. (1959). *Managing for results.* New York: Harper & Row.
Gawain, S. (1978). *Creative visualization.* New York: Bantam Books.
Gellerman, S.W. (1963). *Motivation and productivity.* New York: American Management Association.
Harris, T.A. (1973). *I'm ok, you're ok.* New York: Harper & Row.
Hyatt, C., & Gottlieb, L. (1987). *When smart people fail.* New York: Simon & Shuster.
Kushner, H. (1986). *When all you ever wanted isn't enough.* New York: Simon & Schuster.

Lawler, E.E., III. (1973). *Motivation in work organizations*. Monterey, Calif.: Brooks/Cole.

MacKenzie, R.A. (1972). *The time trap*. New York: McGraw-Hill.

Maltz, M. (1960). *Psychocybernetics*. Englewood Cliffs, N.J.: Prentice-Hall.

Packard, V. (1959). *The status seekers*. New York: David McKay.

Peters, T. (1987). *Thriving on chaos*. New York: Alfred A. Knopf.

Peters, T.J., & Waterman, R.H. (1982). *In search of excellence*. New York: Harper & Row.

Pascarella, P. (1984). *The new achievers*. New York: Macmillan.

Reisman, D. (1950). *The lonely crowd*. New Haven, Conn.: Yale University Press.

Uris, A. (1974). *Thank God it's Monday*. New York: Thomas Y. Crowell.

Whyte, W. (Ed.) (1955). *Money and motivation*. New York: Harper & Row.

Whyte, W. (1956). *The organization man*. New York: Simon & Schuster.

Teaching Staff

9

Objectives

After completing this chapter, you should be able to:

1. Discuss the role of the staff nurse in teaching other staff.
2. Identify principles related to teaching adults.
3. List the steps involved in the teaching process.
4. Describe and give examples of three types of learning.
5. Discuss factors impacting the teaching process.
6. State identified goals for learning in behavioral terms.
7. Match selected teaching strategies with identified objectives.
8. Discuss methods for determining the effectiveness of teaching.
9. Identify possible solutions for problems occurring in staff teaching.

All good nurses are teachers. Nurses teach not only patients and families but also other nursing staff members and sometimes each other. Teaching other nursing personnel is often overlooked as a major responsibility of the staff nurse. Some staff nurses feel that staff teaching is the responsibility of the staff development or inservice education department. In fact, however, the staff nurse is frequently required to teach staff. For example, staff nurses may teach new staff about unit routines and procedures. The staff nurse may also teach staff about dealing with an unusual patient care problem.

Staff teaching may involve informal or spontaneous incidents as well as formal, structured presentations. Informal situations occur during the day-to-day routine of providing patient care. This chapter includes discussions of both types of teaching but focuses primarily on the informal type of teaching.

A SYSTEMATIC APPROACH TO STAFF TEACHING

Regardless of the type of teaching, formal or informal, the process of teaching is systematic and proceeds in a very purposeful manner. The process of teaching, as you probably already know from experience with patient teaching, is similar to the process of patient care. It begins with assessment and planning, moves on to the implementation phase, and ends with an evaluation of the effectiveness of the plan. Similarly, teaching staff is based on certain specific principles and is influenced by a variety of factors.

As a prelude to the discussion of the process of staff teaching, consider the following situations in which teaching is indicated.

Situation 1. A newly employed licensed practical nurse (LPN) asks the staff nurse for help with tracheostomy care and suctioning on Mr. M, a patient who recently had a laryngectomy.

Situation 2. As a staff nurse assists the nursing assistant in transferring Mrs. B from chair to bed, the nurse notices that the assistant uses very poor body mechanics. This nursing assistant frequently complains of back pain.

Situation 3. A student nurse asks the staff nurse to explain exactly what is meant by the order "Bed rest with bathroom privileges." She also asks how this differs from the order "Up ad lib."

Situation 4. During morning report, a staff nurse says, "What does the nursing diagnosis 'ineffective coping' really mean? I think we are using it incorrectly or inappropriately." Another staff member says to the team leader, "Why don't you plan a staff development program for us about nursing diagnosis?"

Situation 5. During a patient care conference, staff members complain that Mrs. C's family is "really getting in the way." They say, "They try to do everything." Mrs. C has recently suffered a stroke, leaving her with left-sided paralysis. Her family plans to take her home following discharge.

These situations are just a few of the "teachable moments" that occur every day on most nursing units. What is a teachable moment? It occurs when there is a felt need for additional information. This need may arise from the environment or situation, such as in situations 2 and 5. Or the need may arise from the learner, as in situations 1, 3, and 4.

How does the staff nurse take the best advantage of the teachable moment? Remember, staff teaching is similar to patient teaching; therefore, the principles guiding nursing actions will also be similar.

Assumptions Related to Adult Education

Knowles (1980) has identified three basic assumptions related to adult education. The first is related to the adult learner's potential for learning. Adults can and will learn. They, in fact, have a natural potential for learning.

Another important assumption is that learning is an individual experience and the center of the experience is internal, not external to the individual. This means that no one can make anyone learn if the individual is not ready or does not want to learn. This assumption mandates the role of the teacher as that of helper or facilitator of learning. The teacher works with the learner to achieve goals and objectives that the learner sees as important.

The third assumption that Knowles identifies is that there are certain conditions that are particularly supportive to the adult learning process. These conditions are listed in the accompanying display. The following discussion presents some principles of teaching and learning that reflect these conditions of learning.

Principles of Teaching and Learning

Adults learn best what they want to know or perceive as being meaningful to their work or personal life. If a person wants to learn how to cross-stitch or give an injection, the experience, although difficult, will also be enjoyable. However, if the individual has no desire to learn to cross-stitch or give an injection, attempts to learn (as well as teach) will most likely become abysmal failures.

The learner must actively participate in the teaching–learning process if learning is to take place. Therefore, any teaching activity must provide

---

Conditions of Learning

The learner

- feels a need to learn.
- perceives the goals of learning to be his/her goals.
- accepts a share of the responsibility of planning and implementing the learning experience.
- experiences a feeling of commitment to learning.
- participates actively in learning.
- experiences a sense of progress towards goals.

The learning environment is characterized by

- physical comfort.
- mutual trust and respect.
- a feeling of mutual helpfulness.
- freedom of expression.
- acceptance of differences.

The learning process

- relates to previous experience of the learner.
- makes sense to the learner.
- provides a sense of progress.

(Adapted from Knowles, M.S. [1980]. *The Modern Practice of Adult Education*. Chicago: Associated Press.)

---

ample opportunity for the learner to participate. The learner should have an opportunity to participate at all levels in the process, including the assessment and planning phase and the implementation phase. The learner should be included in determining the expected learning outcomes and methods used to measure outcomes.

Learning is easier when it is related to what the learner already knows. Therefore, the teacher should begin with what the learner already knows. For example, if a diabetic patient wants to know how to use the exchange system when eating in restaurants, the nurse teaching the patient would relate this to what the patient already knows about planning meals at home using the exchange system.

Learning is retained longer when it is put to immediate use and when it is reinforced. Nothing motivates one to learn like success. Being able to use learning immediately not only promotes retention but also gives the learner a feeling of success. The satisfaction from being able to accomplish the task also reinforces the learning.

Teaching is an interpersonal process. It is a relationship that occurs between two people. Therefore, the emotional climate is important to the learning process. Mutual respect and rapport make the learning process easier. Good communication techniques are essential for establishing rapport, working through the teaching–learning process, and providing appropriate feedback and reinforcement.

THE PROCESS OF TEACHING

Assessment and Planning

The process of teaching includes the same steps as the nursing process, so there are no new steps to memorize. The first step is assessment. This involves gathering information about what needs to be taught as well as factors that will affect the process of learning.

Using the example given in Situation 1, relating to tracheostomy suctioning, let us work through the process of assessment. In this informal teaching setting, the assessment will be done rather quickly and "on the spot." As you recall from patient teaching, it is important to start with what the patient already knows and with what the patient wants to know. The same is true when teaching staff. Adults have a great deal of experience that provides an excellent basis for future learning. Building on experience is important in staff teaching.

In this situation, you can "begin with what the learner already knows" by asking the LPN several questions. For example, asking, "What experience have you had caring for patients with tracheostomies?" will give you information about previous experience with this type of patient. Suppose the LPN indicates that he or she has never had an experience with a patient having a tracheostomy. Then you may need to find out if he or she has ever performed oropharyngeal suctioning. You should also assess her understanding and use of sterile technique.

During the process of assessment, remember to create an environment of acceptance of the learner's need to know. If, for example, you replied to the LPN by saying, "You mean you have never cared for anyone with a trach?" the LPN might feel intimidated and belittled. Acceptance would be communicated by indicating your willingness to work with the LPN in learning this skill.

During the assessment phase, the nurse should also consider any other factors that may influence learning. This includes the learner's physical and mental readiness for learning. The nurse may also consider the learner's level of anxiety as well as other factors such as fatigue, distracting influences, or immediate work agenda.

The next step in the teaching process is planning. Planning includes identifying goals or objectives of teaching and identifying a plan to meet the learning need and goals. The following display provides an illustration

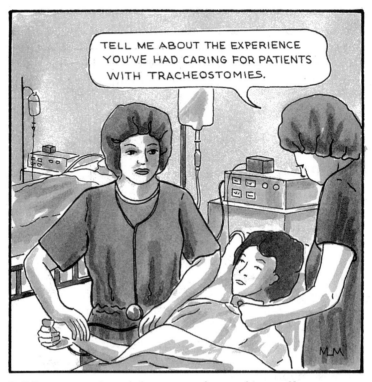

Building on experience is important when teaching staff.

of an "on-the-spot" assessment and planning interaction between the staff nurse and the LPN.

An Assessment-Planning Interaction

RN: Tell me about your experiences related to trach care and suctioning. (The nurse is attempting to build on previous experience.)

LPN: Well, when I was in school, I helped take care of a patient who had a trach but I didn't do any trach care or suctioning.

RN: Were you able to observe anyone performing trach care or suctioning? (The nurse continues the assessment of prior experience.)

LPN: No, I didn't . . . .

RN: That's OK. Now, have you ever done any oropharyngeal suctioning or observed anyone doing this? (The nurse continues to determine level of learner's previous knowledge as well as maintaining an attitude of acceptance of the learner.)

(continued)

An Assessment-Planning Interaction (*Continued*)

LPN: Oh, gee, I haven't done that either. Boy, I don't know anything, do I?

RN: That's OK, too. Patients who have trachs aren't that common in some hospitals. Let's consider some other area. Tell me what you know about trachs in general. What are they, why do patients need to have tracheostomies? (The nurse supplies reasonable rationale for lack of experience, thus demonstrating an attitude of acceptance. The nurse continues assessment.)

LPN: Well, I do know that a tracheostomy is a permanent opening into the trachea and it is usually done because of some kind of obstruction in the laryngeal or upper airway area.

RN: That's very good. Now let's begin with that knowledge. Tell me what you know about sterile technique. (The nurse provides appropriate reinforcement and encouragement.)

LPN: Oh, I've done lots of sterile dressing changes; I know how to correctly put on gloves and I know what's sterile and not sterile. You know I used to work in OR.

RN: I didn't know you worked in OR, that's very good experience. Now, let's get a clear idea of what you want to do. You want to be able to correctly suction Mr. M's trach; and you want to be able to change the dressing around the trach, change the straps on the trach and clean the inner cannula. Is that correct? (The nurse focuses on individual accomplishments. The nurse validates learning objectives with the learner. Identified objectives include action verbs which can be observed.)

LPN: Yes . . . but that seems like a lot to learn at one time.

RN: Yes, it is. So we will break it down into several sessions. First, we'll concentrate on suctioning. Then we'll work on the other. (The nurse listens and responds to learner's concerns.)

LPN: That sounds better, I think I can handle that.

RN: Here's our plan. Mr. M has to be suctioned about every hour. I just did it about 10 minutes ago, so it will probably need to be done again at about 10:00 A.M. Between now and then, why don't you read over the procedure in the manual. Bring the manual with you to the room, and I will suction him and go over each step in the procedure. You can ask questions. After that, you can practice the technique using a glass of water to simulate the suctioning. I will watch and make suggestions. Then, if you feel ready, you can suction him at 11:00 A.M. while I watch and assist you as needed. (The nurse reveals a specific plan for the learner's approval and outlines responsibilities of both the teacher and the learner. The nurse provides an opportunity to practice in a nonthreatening environment.)

LPN: Sounds great! I really appreciate your help.

Types of Learning

The type of learning that is to occur should be considered during the planning process. There are three types of learning: cognitive, psychomotor, and affective. *Cognitive* learning involves learning facts and knowledge. Some examples of cognitive learning are being able to name the 12 cranial nerves, listing the signs and symptoms of hemorrhagic shock, and identifying the drug classification of morphine.

Psychomotor learning involves learning how to do something, such as giving injections, starting an intravenous line, and transferring the patient from the bed to a chair. It involves learning facts as well as doing something with your hands or body.

The third type is *affective* learning, which involves attitudes, values, and feelings. This type of learning occurs gradually and perhaps unconsciously. Values and attitudes are difficult to change and even more difficult to measure. However, this type of learning is often necessary if the nursing staff wishes to provide high-quality nursing care. Some examples of affective learning include acceptance of certain ethnic minority groups' and allegiance to a political party or religious group. It might also include your idea of the ideal nurse.

Why is it important to identify the type of learning? The type of learning determines how you will teach as well as how you will evaluate whether learning has occurred. Let us go back to Situation 1. What type of learning should occur in this situation? Obviously, this is an example of psychomotor learning. The LPN needs to learn *how to do* tracheostomy care and suctioning. If psychomotor learning is to occur, then simply talking about how to do the procedure will probably not accomplish the identified goals. Although reading about the procedure in the hospital manual is helpful, this is not all that is needed if the learner is to accomplish the goal of *doing* tracheostomy care and suctioning. In addition to providing facts and knowledge about how to do tracheostomy care, the nurse should provide a step-by-step demonstration of tracheostomy care and suctioning and an opportunity for the LPN to practice the skill.

The type of learning also assists in evaluating the effectiveness of the teaching–learning activity. For example, when determining the effectiveness of the activity, you would expect that the LPN would be able to demonstrate appropriate technique when providing tracheostomy care for the patient.

Identifying Goals

Another important part of the planning phase is identifying clear, attainable goals. Well-stated goals and objectives for teaching are just as essential as well-stated diagnoses and goals in planning patient care. Both give the nurse a clear direction for action and indicate when the goals have been met.

Consider Situation 4—the situation related to the staff's questions about nursing diagnosis. In this situation, where assessment and planning become very important, a formal teaching session may be more appropriate than informal teaching. First, from the information presented, it is difficult to determine exactly what the members of the staff are interested in learning. Do they want more information about ineffective coping or information about nursing diagnoses in general? Or is this perhaps a type of affective learning? Are they questioning whether nursing diagnoses in general are helpful for nurses to use? An astute nurse, intent on seizing the teachable moment, will attempt to get as much information as possible before he or she proceeds in the teaching process.

Suppose, after a period of assessment, the nurse and staff members decide that more information is needed about the nursing diagnosis of ineffective coping. The nurse identifies the following goals for the presentation.

Following an inservice presentation about the nursing diagnosis of ineffective coping, the staff will be able to
- List the defining characteristics of ineffective coping.
- Identify possible etiologic or contributing factors.
- Write a nursing diagnosis for ineffective coping using correct Problem–Etiology–Signs and Symptoms (P–E–S) format.

One characteristic of a clearly stated objective is the identification of *who* will be learning and *under what conditions*. In this example, the staff members are those involved in learning and the conditions are "following an inservice presentation. . . . " Another characteristic is that behavior is stated in action verbs that can be observed. For example, the staff nurse will be able to observe if the staff can "list," "identify," and "write." Suppose the nurse identified this objective, "Know the etiologic factors related to ineffective coping." Could she observe knowing? No, that is impossible.

Well-stated objectives should also include any standards used for evaluation. Objective C provides an example of standards. The standard is "using correct P–E–S format." This standard provides additional information to both the learner and the teacher about the quality of the outcome.

These objectives assist the nurse in identifying the information that needs to be presented to the group and providing guidelines for determining the effectiveness of the teaching activity. Prior to making the presentation, the nurse should share these objectives with the group to be certain that the staff members agree on the identified outcomes.

Planning the Content

Using the objectives listed earlier, the staff nurse could easily plan the formal presentation. An outline for the presentation would include the following:

1. Definition and defining characteristics of ineffective coping
2. Etiologic factors related to ineffective coping
3. Signs and symptoms indicative of ineffective coping
4. Time to practice writing a nursing diagnostic statement

Because one of the objectives involves actually writing a nursing diagnosis for a patient experiencing ineffective coping, the staff nurse must include time for the staff to do so.

Planning the Strategy

Selecting teaching strategies is an important part of the planning phase. Many strategies are useful in presenting material as well as demonstrating skills. One of the most frequently used teaching strategies is the lecture approach, which involves "telling" the audience about the concept to be studied. This particular approach requires little participation from the audience. For that reason the staff nurse may want to consider other approaches that will encourage more participation.

One approach that might be used is that of the case study. The staff nurse could present information about a patient who has been diagnosed as experiencing ineffective coping. Then specific information about the diagnosis could be applied to this patient situation. It really does not matter, for the sake of learning, whether the diagnosis has been correctly made. The staff should be able to meet the objectives of the presentation regardless.

Games are another interesting teaching strategy. Dols (1988) presents an interesting strategy for teaching nursing diagnosis using a card game.

Another approach is a poster presentation. The staff nurse could construct colorful and interesting posters containing the information related to ineffective coping. The posters could be placed in a conspicuous area, convenient for all staff. If the posters are available prior to the presentation, the staff nurse could quickly review the information and move directly to the actual writing of the diagnostic statement. Poster presentations are effective ways to present information about a variety of subjects, such as new drugs, unfamiliar medical diagnoses, or new procedures. Figure 9-1 illustrates a poster presentation related to a new medication. The advantage of this approach is the effective use of time and individual participation in the process. The disadvantages include the time needed to prepare effective presentations.

DRUG: Terramycin

CLASSIFICATION Anti infective; Antibiotic

DOSAGE & ROUTE OF ADMINISTRATION

Adult: PO: 250–500 mgm q 6–12h

IM: 100 mgm q 8–12h up to 250 mgm

IV: 250–500 mgm q 12h (Do not exceed 500 mgm q 6h)

SIDE EFFECTS & TOXIC EFFECTS

Nausea, vomiting, diarrhea, stomatitis;
Skin rash, superinfections,
Renal toxicity

**Pregnancy-category D-positive evidence of human fetal risk

NURSING IMPLICATIONS & PATIENT TEACHING

- Check expiration date
- Adm PO at 1 hour before or 2 hours after meals
- Avoid exposure to sunlight
- Do not give with milk, milk products, antacids, or calcium containing foods.

Figure 9-1. Poster presentation on new medication.

Filmstrips, movies, and video tapes are another effective way to present information and to teach skills. These media presentations can be used for large group presentations or individual viewing. To be certain that the material matches the objectives of the activity, filmstrips and other media should be previewed prior to showing.

Demonstrations are the most useful method for teaching psychomotor skills. The demonstrator should emphasize the major steps in the process, as well as critical processes, especially those related to patient and staff safety. Videotapes and movies may also be used to demonstrate skills. Filmstrips are usually less successful, because they do not show the actual movements that are critical to achieving psychomotor skills.

Implementation

The implementation phase involves actually putting the plan into action. During this phase it is important to remember that teaching is an interpersonal process and that a comfortable climate helps to create an atmosphere of mutual trust in which the learner feels free to ask questions without feeling foolish. The teacher is responsible for establishing this atmosphere of trust. The staff nurse can encourage feelings of trust by maintaining structure, setting limits, and giving appropriate, supportive feedback. The staff nurse provides structure by providing a road map for learning. This road map includes a clear identification of goals and objectives and a clear understanding of the responsibilities of the both the teacher and the learner. Look at the structure provided in the "Assessment—Planning Interaction" display (p. 204). The staff nurse specifically outlines responsibilities for himself or herself and the LPN. Providing structures does not mean that the teacher is inflexible. Good structure provides for individual differences.

Feedback is extremely important during the implementation phase. It assists the learner by reinforcing appropriate behavior. If the staff nurse intends to foster an environment of questioning, responding positively to all questions is essential. The nurse may initially respond to questions by saying, "That's a good question. Let's talk about it for a minute." If learners ask questions that are unrelated to the topic being discussed, the nurse needs to decide how to respond without squelching the learner's need to know. The nurse may respond by saying, "That's a good question. Could we discuss it at the end of the session?"

A comfortable physical environment is also important to consider during the implementation phase. Prior to a structured group presentation, the nurse should consider the comfort of the seating arrangement, the temperature in the room, and other environmental factors such as noise and possible interruptions.

Timing for implementation is also important. Group learning should be scheduled when most of the staff can attend. Scheduling teaching at the beginning or the end of the shift may not be the most appropriate time because staff may be anxious to begin or get off work. When implementing individual teaching, be sure to consider other tasks the individual may be trying to accomplish. For example, expecting the staff to learn something new when they feel rushed and overworked may lead to frustration of both the teacher and the staff.

During the implementation phase, the nurse should make sure teaching materials being used are appropriate for use in the given teaching setting. Nothing is more frustrating than trying to look at a handout with someone else or trying to read overhead transparencies that are poorly made and difficult to read. Make sure there are adequate handouts for all participants. Likewise, be sure that other teaching materials can easily be seen by all participants.

Lastly, remember the old adage "That which is learned with laughter is learned well." If you can add some humor to your teaching, do it. This does not mean that you do not take the learning situation seriously; it does mean, however, that you take the responsibility of establishing a joyful learning situation just as seriously. Use cartoons, jokes, or funny stories to illustrate your point, if possible.

Evaluation

The evaluation phase is extremely important and may never be overlooked. A good plan is identified and implemented but never evaluated. Just as there are numerous strategies for teaching, there are many ways to evaluate learning. Psychomotor learning obviously needs to be evaluated in terms of the learner's ability to perform some new skill consistently. In Situation 1 the LPN should be able to suction the patient correctly every time, and without supervision. In Situation 2 the nursing assistant should be able to transfer patients consistently, using appropriate body mechanics.

Cognitive learning can be evaluated using a variety of techniques. In Situation 4 the staff nurse could wait a period of 2 to 3 weeks, then evaluate the effectiveness of teaching by surveying nursing care plans to determine if the nursing diagnosis "ineffective coping" is being used appropriately.

The nurse may also administer a brief post-test at the end of the session or at a later date. Because "tests" are threatening to many individuals, every effort should be made to make this experience as nonthreatening as possible. This can be done in several ways. One might be to have participants complete the test anonymously. Another is to have at least two, or more, participants complete one test as a group. The test could be administered and then answers could be given so that participants could assess their own progress.

Lastly, the teacher and the learner should remember that evaluation is just one more part of the cycle of learning. Evaluation provides guidelines for continued improvement, not retribution. Evaluation should be looked upon as a kind of reassessment in which strengths and areas for improvements are identified.

PROBLEM AREAS IN STAFF TEACHING

As with many other management responsibilities, staff teaching also can present some challenges and concerns. Being aware of the more commonly occurring problems will put you in a position to more effectively meet them.

Encouraging Awareness of Learning Needs

One situation that may be problematic for the staff nurse as teacher is one in which the situation indicates a need for learning and in which the learner may be unaware of the need. This problem occurs in situations 2 and 5. In the first situation related to the nursing assistant's poor body mechanics, the need to learn is not obvious to the assistant. The role of nurse as a facilitator of learning becomes much more important. It is the nurse's responsibility to help the learner identify the problem. How can the staff nurse do this?

Consider the following approaches:

Approach 1. The staff nurse says to the assistant, "I noticed that you used very poor body mechanics when assisting Mr. B back to bed. Do you think that could be the cause of all the back pain you've been having?"

Approach 2. The nurse says, "I noticed when you were assisting Mrs. B back to bed, you winced several times as if you were having some difficulty. Have you been experiencing any other problems lifting and moving patients?"

The second approach, in which the nurse relates what she has observed to the learner and asks for validation as well as any other information the assistant may have to offer, is obviously better than the first. This approach will encourage the learner to explore some possible causes of the difficulty and may initiate a need to learn on the part of the learner. The second approach is less blame directed and more supportive of the staff. Remember, learning occurs more easily if the learner is aware of the need to learn and if the material to be learned is directly related to improvement of the learner's work or personal life. The second approach also permits the nurse to gather more data before drawing conclusions.

Now let us consider Situation 5. In this situation staff members complain that a patient's family is "in the way" because they want to do everything for the patient. The patient is recovering from a CVA and has left-sided paralysis. The nurse's role as facilitator of learning becomes more complex. The type of learning in this situation is affective learning. As you recall, affective learning deals with values, attitudes, and personal preferences. The staff in this situation needs to become more open to the needs of the family.

Affective learning involves several processes, the first of which is awareness. In the beginning, the learner may simply become aware of something. In the movie *Dead Poets' Society* the teacher stands on the top of his desk (and has the students do so as well) to illustrate a technique of looking at things from a different perspective. If the staff nurse wants to increase awareness, he or she may have to arrange an incident in which the staff looks at the situation from a different angle. Consider these approaches by the nurse:

> *Approach 1.* The nurse replies to the staff, "Come on, all of you know Mrs. C's family has been so attentive. Why don't you just let them do whatever they can do and then you do the rest? You know they will be taking care of her when she goes home anyway."
>
> *Approach 2.* The nurse replies, "I have noticed that you seem to be particularly frustrated dealing with Mrs. C and her family. Can we schedule a patient care conference to discuss ways to deal with the family?"
>
> *Approach 3.* The nurse replies, "Working with Mrs. C and her family does seem to be particularly frustrating. The family is planning to care for her when she goes home, aren't they? Maybe that makes our

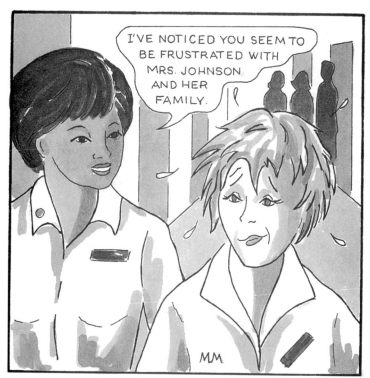

It is the nurse's responsibility to help the learner identify the problem.

role a little different. Do you think that perhaps they see us as supervisors of their care rather than as actual caregivers?"

The first approach obviously destroys the teachable moment. The nurse does not respond to the needs of the staff or the patient and her family. The second approach is somewhat better, although no attention has been given to the need to encourage the staff's awareness. Perhaps the nurse intends to do this in the patient care conference.

The third approach is the best. First the nurse acknowledges and accepts the staff's frustration. Then, without chastisement, the nurse provides an opportunity for the staff to consider Mrs. C and her family from a different angle. Other approaches include using "What if . . ." statements. The nurse could say to the staff, "What if the family really does want to do everything for Mrs. C?" The nurse might also pose this question, "What if we were Mrs. C's daughters? What would we want from the staff?"

Affective learning occurs at a different rate from cognitive and psychomotor learning. Thus, the nurse must be patient and tolerant of the staff's need to move more slowly. The situation with Mrs. C provides an excellent situation to teach by example. The staff nurse may elect to work directly with Mrs. C's family, allowing them to take the lead in the care of the patient, while the nurse functions in the role of supervisor of that care. This type of teaching is referred to as role modeling.

Finding Time to Teach

A perpetual problem in nursing is finding time to do all the things that a nurse is expected to do. Finding time to teach is no exception. How long does it take to work through the process of teaching? Go back and read through the "Assessment—Planning Interaction" (p. 204), or have a classmate role-play this situation with you. That entire interaction lasts about 2 minutes and 15 seconds. What additional time will be needed on the part of the staff nurse? Other than supervising the simulated practice, the nurse will actually be doing procedures she would be doing anyway, so the additional time needed to teach the LPN this skill is minimal.

Nurses seem to find time to do those things they consider important. So one solution to the problem may lie in the staff nurse's assessment of the importance of different functions that must be accomplished. The "bottom line" is a determination of what is best for patients. Meeting the staff's need for learning and growth adds to their job satisfaction. More satisfied employees add significantly to the quality of life on a nursing unit and the quality of care provided.

Remember that teaching, like other aspects of nursing, becomes easier and more efficiently implemented with time and experience. To the staff nurse concerned with the need to teach, seizing the teachable moment soon becomes almost automatic.

Staff Members Who Appear to Resist Learning

Staff nurses are occasionally confronted with an individual who appears to resist learning. The first step in dealing with this type of learner is, of course, assessment. The nurse should seek answers to questions such as, "Is there some reason this individual seems to resist teaching?" or, "Is there something else going on in this person's life that is interfering with the ability to learn?" Adult education experts assert that all adults want to learn. Therefore, when faced with the situation of a person who does not appear to want to learn, other factors should be considered.

Earlier in this chapter the relationship of success and learning was discussed. When working with the difficult learner the nurse might explore ways to provide a feeling of success. The astute nurse will seek opportunities to provide positive feedback to the employee who seems to resist learning. Additionally, the nurse will watch for clues about other factors. For example, the nurse will listen for clues about the employee's job satisfaction and the employee's perception of possibilities for advancement. Employees who see no future advancement opportunities may view learning in a very negative light.

Other factors that should be considered when facing the problem of the seemingly resistant learner include personal problems, previous learning experiences, and capabilities of the learner. Overwhelming personal problems may interfere with the employee's ability to learn. Remember, defining the term *overwhelming* rests with the individual involved in the problem, not the onlooker. Severe anxiety also limits an individual's ability to pay attention and learn.

Previous learning experiences are important to consider in determining possible reasons for the behavior of the resistant learner. Past learning experiences that were characteristically painful, frustrating, or embarrassing have tremendous influence on the individual's desire to seek new learning experiences. Providing a learning environment that is non-threatening and supportive would be an important intervention with this particular learner.

Another factor to consider is the resistant learner's actual capacity to learn. If the learner has limited or nonexistent reading abilities, then teaching strategies that involve reading will be seen as threatening experiences to be avoided. The nurse can assess learning abilities on a day-to-day basis when working with other nursing staff. Providing other methods of learning, such as filmstrips, demonstrations, or lectures would be more appropriate for the employee who has difficulty reading.

SUMMARY

Teaching nursing staff personnel is a major function of the staff nurse. This teaching may be formal or informal, with much of it occurring during the day-to-day routine of providing quality patient care.

The teaching of staff is based on several assumptions related to adult education: (1) Adults can and will learn; (2) adults want to learn; (3) learning is an internal individual experience; (4) certain conditions are particularly conducive to learning.

The process of teaching is systematic and purposeful. It proceeds in an orderly manner, beginning with assessment; moves to planning and implementation; and ends with evaluation. The process of teaching is guided by principles related to adult education.

Adults learn best what they want to know and what they perceive to be important. Active participation on the part of the learner is necessary for learning to take place. Learning is easier when it is related to what the learner already knows. Learning is retained longer when it is put to immediate use. Reinforcement enhances learning. Teaching is an interpersonal process that occurs best in a climate of trust and acceptance.

The process of assessment involves gathering information about what needs to be taught, creating an environment of trust, and the consideration of factors influencing the teaching–learning process.

During the planning phase the nurse and learner identify goals and objectives. These objectives provide directions for implementation and evaluation. The three types of learning—cognitive, psychomotor, and affective—should be considered during the planning phase. Types of learning dictate methods of teaching and evaluation. A variety of teaching strategies can be used to meet identified objectives. Some of these are lectures, discussions, demonstrations, poster presentations, games, and case studies.

Establishing an environment of trust is important during the implementation phase. The nurse should consider physical and emotional factors in the environment. During the implementation phase, feedback is important to enhance learning.

Evaluation is an integral part of the teaching process. It involves a reassessment of learning goals and objectives.

Problem areas in staff teaching include increasing learners' awareness of learning needs, finding time to teach, and working with the reticent learner.

Study Questions/Activities

1. From your past experience identify several situations in which you observed a staff nurse teaching staff.
2. Give several examples of cognitive, psychomotor, and affective learning other than the ones listed in this chapter.
3. A new nursing assistant asked you to help her learn how to take an apical pulse. What would you do first?
4. Write a clearly stated objective for each of the following learning needs:
   a. A younger student asks you to tell her how to recognize early signs of oxygen deprivation.
   b. A licensed practical nurse asks about the side-effects of the antidepressant Elavil.
   c. A nursing assistant asks you how to measure a patient's urinary output.
5. For each of the situations in the preceding question identify at least one teaching strategy to meet your identified objectives.
6. Identify several methods for evaluating outcomes in each of the situations in question 4.
7. Talk to several staff nurses. Ask them what kinds of problems they have encountered when teaching staff.

REFERENCES

Dols, J.D. (1988). An innovative strategy for teaching care plan writing. *The Journal of Continuing Education in Nursing, 19*(3), 131–133.

Knowles, M.S. (1980). *The modern practice of adult education: Revised and updated.* Chicago: Association Press.

SUGGESTIONS FOR FURTHER READING

Binger, J.L., & Huntsman, A.J. (1988). Coaching: A technique to increase employee performance. *AORN Journal, 47*(1), 229, 232–233, 235, 237.

Hast, A.S. (1987). Self-learning packages in critical care. *Critical Care Nurse, 7*(2), 110–116.

Lawler, T.G. (1988). The objectives of performance appraisal—or "Where do we go from here?" *Nursing Management, 19*(3), 82–84, 86, 88,

Lewis, D.J. (1989). Gaming: A teaching strategy for adult learners. *Journal of Continuing Education in Nursing, 20*(2), 80–84.

Sheehy, S.B. (1987). Ways to present clinical topics. *Journal of Emergency Nursing, 13*(6), 377–379.

Shelton, S.E. (1988). Keeping pace with nursing literature through a professional gerontological nursing journal club. *Journal of Gerontological Nursing, 14*(11), 26–28.

Smith, C.E. (1978). Planning, implementing and evaluating learning experiences for adults. *Nurse Educator, 3*(6), 31–36.

Stearns, N.S., Ottoson, J.M., & Haitz, M.C. (1985). Literature on the go. *American Journal of Nursing, 85*(10), 1161–1162.

Tarnow, K.G. (1979). Working with adult learners. *Nurse Educator, 4*(5), 34–40.

Wilkinson, J. (1989). Role modeling as a teaching strategy. *AD Nurse, 4*(1), 29–32.

Williams, J. (1986). The mobile educational crash cart: Self-directed learning supplement that meets staff needs. *Journal of Continuing Education in Nursing, 17*(2), 59–61.

Developing Management Skills

III

The last unit of study in this text deals with topics that you might place in a category related to the skills of management. Exploring effective techniques of receiving and providing feedback gives basic understanding for the more formal performance evaluation system and offers timely tips on managing those responsibilities. Looking at approaches to conflict management and resolution gives you an important perspective as you walk into a new employment environment. Identifying and using your skills as an advocate may be critical to your effectiveness as a new graduate. And being able to understand and apply basic principles of research to your beginning practice may make a difference in how effective your care will be. This text concludes with these various skill aspects of the nurse's role as manager and coordinator of nursing care.

Providing Feedback and Evaluation

Objectives

After completing this chapter, you should be able to:

10

1. Identify the components of the communication process.
2. Discuss verbal and nonverbal skills important to feedback and evaluation.
3. Define positive and negative feedback and give examples of each.
4. List at least five guidelines to be observed when providing both positive and negative feedback.
5. Discuss the purposes of performance appraisal from the perspective of the employee and the organization.
6. Identify three characteristics of an effective performance evaluation system.
7. Identify several types of performance evaluation tools and discuss the advantages and disadvantages of each. These tools include narrative technique, rating scales, checklist, and management by objectives.
8. Discuss the importance of avoiding rater bias and identify some tools used for that purpose.
9. Explain how the timing of a performance appraisal interview and the place in which it is conducted may affect the outcome.
10. Outline factors to consider when conducting a performance appraisal interview.
11. Describe why feedback is critical to evaluation.
12. Identify the purpose of progressive discipline and outline the steps to be followed.
13. Discuss critical elements to be considered when dealing with progressive discipline.
14. List guiding questions concerning progressive discipline.

Of all the topics discussed in this text, the one with which you may have had the most experience involves feedback and evaluation. Feedback, both informal and formal, on how we are performing surrounds us from the time we are born, through elementary and secondary school, into college, and on to the job. You have known this process informally as words of encouragement and direction from your parents as you learned to walk and talk and as they directed you toward abiding by social norms. The report cards and end-of-the-semester evaluations you received in elementary and secondary school are examples of more formal application of evaluation. You have encountered, and will continue to encounter, it in your work environment. As you grow professionally, you may also find yourself in the position of evaluating the performance of others.

In this chapter we shall discuss both formal and informal feedback. One aspect of the formal process of feedback is that of performance appraisal. We shall outline the purposes and goals of performance evaluation and relate the feedback system to the entire process. Characteristics of a good performance appraisal system will be presented and different types of tools that can be used in the process will be discussed briefly. We shall also review some of the pitfalls encountered in the process. A brief discussion of progressive discipline will conclude the chapter.

PROVIDING FEEDBACK

Central to working effectively in a management role is the ability of the manager to communicate skillfully. Entire books are written and semester-long classes are conducted on the topic of organizational communication. Here you will discover how communication skills can be applied to leadership—for example, how blocking ideas or controlling the process of events supports authoritarian management styles or how seeking ideas or facilitating group process encourages participative management.

Reviewing the Communication Process

Undoubtedly, you have had a course on the basics of communication, or the relevant content was integrated into your other courses. In those classes you learned communication terms such as *sender* and *receiver, encode* and *decode, message* and *feedback*. You learned that encoding is the process by which the sender's ideas are converted into the message and that decoding is the process by which the receiver interprets the message sent. Feedback includes a mechanism by which the sender can obtain reactions from the receiver to determine how the message was received. Did the receiver understand the message? Was he or she upset with it? Did he or she agree with it?

Various types of feedback can be used to obtain these answers. Feedback can be direct (*i.e.,* face-to-face exchange), or it can be indirect (*i.e.,* written in a memorandum). It can also be external, as when the listener responds to our message, or it can be internal, as occurs when we know we spoke harshly or angrily. All these types of feedback are used in carrying out nursing activities.

Developing Effective Feedback Techniques

As you move into the role of a registered nurse in which you are responsible for guiding and directing the actions of others, you will find that you use all the communications skills you learned in school and will search for additional ones. From your student days you will recall that messages can be both verbal and nonverbal and that our skills in nonverbal communication are as important as the verbal skills we develop.

Verbal Communication

When concentrating on improving one's verbal communication we need to remember that words carry different meanings to different people. A typical example is the word *shot,* which to most nurses refers to an injection. To a child this may be associated with the type of shot that comes from a gun and results in death or injury. Therefore, we encourage nurses working with children not to use the word *shot.*

It is also important to remember that our perceptions are always incomplete. Words represent generalized symbols that must leave out unique details in order to be efficient. An example is the message parents often give to their children: "You know perfectly well what I mean," which may not be clear to the child. Because this is a characteristic of language, it is important that we seek feedback regarding the messages we send. Verifying with others that they perceived your communication to be the same as you intended is a critical element in communicating effectively.

Nonverbal Communication

Nonverbal communication is usually referred to as the message we send by our physical appearance and movement. It encompasses a wide variety of elements, including facial expression, physical appearance (*e.g.,* the clothes worn), body language (*e.g.,* postures and gestures), eye contact, and the use of touch. The message transmitted nonverbally may be read much more keenly than the verbal one. We work at developing nonverbal skills to assist us in carrying out our responsibilities. For example, many persons in administrative positions nonverbally communicate that an interview is terminated by rising from behind their desks. The very fact that the interview is conducted by the administrator from behind the desk also sends a message. As you perfect your communication skills you will want to reflect on the message you send nonverbally.

We are also aware that words and other nonverbal forms of communication carry different values in different cultures. Think, for example, of the handshake. It can be firm or it can be a gentle clasp. Some cultures view a firm handshake as connoting sureness, honesty, and forthright behavior. Other cultures would interpret a firm handshake as a symbol of aggressive behavior. Most of us think of the ability to maintain eye contact as an important characteristic. However, in some cultures eye contact may be avoided because it is viewed as brazen and insolent. Casting the eyes downward may be a symbol of respect for this person. When touch is employed in communicating, even greater variables can exist. Some see the use of touch as "reaching out" or literally establishing communication with another such as the pat on the back. Entire approaches have been developed using "therapeutic touch." But some cultures would see the touching of another person, especially without that person's permission,

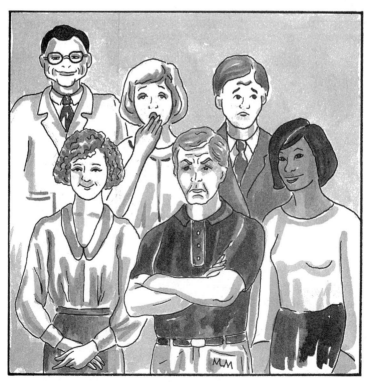

Nonverbal communication encompasses a wide variety of features that include facial expression and postures.

as a serious taboo. Elaborate mechanisms to provide for personal territory free from touch have been developed.

FEEDBACK IN THE WORK ENVIRONMENT

Feedback is important to all of us. Knowing how we are performing, how close we are coming to what is being expected of us, helps maintain motivation. It also helps us to understand the goals of the organization and how we are valued by that organization.

As mentioned earlier, feedback can be both informal and formal. When we talk about informal feedback, we are referring to the kind of information that is provided to us on an hour-to-hour or day-to-day basis. It occurs most frequently as one aspect of the operation of any unit where is it necessary to give direction, help, instructions, reinforcement, or correction to others. We also apply certain adjectives to the word *feedback*. When using it in association with the evaluation process, the most common adjectives are *negative* or *critical* and *positive* or *constructive*.

Guidelines for Providing Positive Feedback

Most persons who are responsible for evaluating the performance of others have little difficulty with positive feedback. If any problem exists, it is usually that positive feedback is not given frequently enough. Because constructive comments help an individual develop self-esteem and provide motivation, the wise and mature manager looks for opportunities to let employees know that their efforts are recognized and appreciated. When the primary nurse says to the licensed practical nurse who is assisting with the care of patients, "Mr. Johansen looked very nice after you finished the morning care," the practical nurse knows that her efforts were noticed and valued. This is referred to by Kron (1981) as a "psychological paycheck." Positive feedback also serves to clarify performance expectations and lets employees know they are "on the right track." All these factors result in greater job satisfaction and better patient care.

Several guidelines can be followed that make positive feedback most effective. It should occur frequently for the reasons we have just mentioned. It should also occur in a timely manner. Saving a positive comment until the next formal interview delays the gratification that it should provide. And, unlike negative feedback, which should always be given in private, positive comments about a person's work often may be given in public. A manager who finds timely occasions to reinforce the good working behaviors of others raises the *esprit de corps* in the area as well as increasing the self-esteem of the person receiving the compliment. Finally, feedback should always be accurate, sincere, and objective.

Responding to Positive Feedback

Some persons are uncomfortable when receiving any type of feedback, especially positive comments. Compliments about your performance, behavior, or professional demeanor should be accepted with dignity. It is appropriate to express your appreciation by a simple and sincere "Thank you." A statement such as, "Thank you for noticing," or, "Thank you; I've been trying to improve that skill," graciously accepts the compliment given.

Guidelines for Providing Negative Feedback

Providing negative feedback is equally important and often more difficult. It is necessary to point out to an employee when he or she is doing something wrong; that is, to correct unsatisfactory performance. It takes skill and experience to develop methods of providing feedback that will help the employee to grow and learn. This is part of the coaching role of a manager and requires that the manager be able to suggest ways to make needed changes. Some managers find it easier to ignore the behavior and do not attempt to correct it. Such managers will eventually discover that not correcting inappropriate behavior frustrates the whole team and lowers staff morale.

When it is necessary to let an employee know that his or her performance must change, some steps can be followed to make this a helpful experience. As with positive feedback, it should be timely and be given as soon as possible after the incident upon which the comment is based. Delaying comment may be construed as approving the unacceptable behavior. Like positive feedback, it should also be frequent, objective, and accurate. If feedback is provided frequently, it becomes less threatening to those receiving it and easier for those giving it. When we say it should be objective and accurate, we mean it should be based directly on observable behaviors rather than on personality traits or personal likes or dislikes. It should include suggestions for change or alternative behaviors and should be appropriately communicated. This means that it should avoid sending put-down or blaming messages. In a similar vein, it should be non-threatening. Highly threatening messages usurp energies that are better spent on improving care than on reducing the threat. Statements such as, "I don't want to see you doing that again," or, "You won't last long if you continue that behavior," are threatening. Remember, all persons are susceptible to feeling threatened. Finally, unlike positive feedback, negative comments should always be given in private.

Responding to Negative Feedback

Initially, as a new graduate you will be receiving evaluative feedback more often than providing it. There may be occasions when you actually seek feedback. Statements such as, "Were my assessments of Mrs. James accurate?" or, "Please check to see that I have programmed this monitor correctly," are asking for feedback. The reasons for seeking feedback are the same as the reasons for providing it. Not surprisingly, then, the skills in receiving feedback are similar to those for providing it.

If you are a conscientious employee, you will give some serious thought to the type of feedback you are receiving. If you find that most of the feedback you are receiving is negative, it may be very difficult to discuss it further. You may feel defensive about the comments that have been made. In such situations it is important that the communications be clarified. Such comments as, "How might I improve my skills?" or, "How can I be of greater assistance?" may be good openers. Restating a message is valuable in determining that you understood what was being said. Statements such as, "What I heard you say was I need to look for opportunities to help others," provide opportunity for verification, clarification, or expansion. Notice that all messages are in the form of "I" statements.

FORMAL PERFORMANCE APPRAISAL

Purposes of a Formal Appraisal

When feedback moves to a more formal structure it is referred to as evaluation or performance appraisal. An effective performance appraisal system has at least two major purposes. The first of these relates to the functioning of the organization; the second refers to the personal development of the employee within the organization. Some would also give a third reason for evaluation: to provide a basis for termination of an employee from a position, should that be necessary.

For the organization, performance appraisal can provide information upon which to base management decisions regarding such matters as salary increases, promotion, transfer, demotion, and termination. The organization may also use this process to target individuals for merit wage increases. Performance appraisal will help assess the effectiveness of hiring and recruiting practices that have been used by the organization. It can also supply information to the organization that will help to identify training and development needs of the employees and, in that way, assist in the structure of staff development programs. Inherent in this process is the establishment of standards of job performance, which also benefits any organization.

Performance appraisals are used to assist employees in their personal development. The employee and the supervisor can develop plans that will result in the personal growth of the employee. This might include increased skill performance, technical training, or a formal advance in education that will help improve future performance. In addition to providing information about a particular individual's performance, the future goals and aspirations of the employee can be identified and made known to management. A performance interview, properly conducted, results in improved communication between the supervisor and the employee. It provides an established opportunity for the supervisor to recognize the accomplishments of the employee. Receiving recognition for a job well done motivates employees to continue doing their best (see Chap. 8).

Some persons, both employees and supervisors, view the evaluation process negatively. For the employee this may be a carryover from earlier associations with evaluation, when it could result in grades and perhaps being told, "You can do better." Supervisors may believe the process is too time-consuming, requiring judgments that they do not believe they have the knowledge or skills to make. Some tend to view this responsibility as "playing God" (McGregor, 1972). Both might be valid if the process is not clearly defined and soundly implemented. Employees need assistance in seeing this as an opportunity for growth, and the supervisors must learn to view this as an opportunity to do a better coaching and counseling job. Both coaching and counseling of subordinates are important aspects of the supervisory role.

Oberg (1972) identified some common problems that interfere with the success of formal appraisal programs. Included were the following:

1. Performance appraisal programs may be viewed as demanding too much from supervisors, in that it is difficult for a first-line supervisor to know what each of 20, 30, or more subordinates is doing.
2. Standards and ratings tend to vary widely, with some raters being tough and others more lenient.
3. An appraiser may replace organizational standards with personal values and bias.
4. Because of lack of communication, standards by which employees think they are being judged are sometimes different from those their superiors actually use.
5. Appraisal techniques tend to be used as performance panaceas and cannot replace sound selection, placement, and training programs.
6. The validity of ratings may be reduced by the supervisor's resistance to making the ratings, because of the discomfort they feel when having to confront the employee with negative ratings and negative feedback.
7. Ratings can boomerang when communicated to employees, be-

cause negative feedback fails to motivate the typical employee and may cause that employee to perform worse.

8. Performance appraisals may interfere with the more constructive coaching relationship between the supervisor and the employee. Supervisors may see the role of evaluator as placing them in the role of judge.

It is important that all persons involved in the evaluation system be aware of these common concerns so that steps can be taken to diminish or eliminate them. All employees need and want to know how they are doing, and a properly conducted evaluation session can effectively provide that information.

Characteristics of an Effective Performance Appraisal System

We can probably all recall some instance in our life when we were unhappy about the way we were evaluated. For some it might have been an experience in which the way the clinical evaluation was done by an instructor or the criteria that were used to conduct it seemed unfair. For others it might have been an actual work situation. In other instances, we can probably all remember an instance in which the review of our performance was conducted so positively that it helped us to move forward professionally and resulted in our respect and admiration for the person who assisted us in that process. What factors must come together to ensure that the evaluation process has a positive outcome? What must occur for everyone to believe it is a meaningful investment of time and energy?

Relating Performance Appraisal to the Job Description

All individuals have a right to know the criteria by which they will be evaluated. These criteria most logically evolve from well-written job descriptions. Like the behavioral objectives that guided your learning as a student, job descriptions should describe what an employee is expected to do in a particular position. As you learned in Chapter 1, job descriptions are written statements describing the responsibilities of each position within the organization. Each organization is composed of many job descriptions that, when reviewed in total, can provide a great deal of information about the structure of any organization. Job descriptions should contain statements that describe the duties and responsibilities for which the employee is responsible. They should include only those characteristics that are important and necessary for successful performance. They should be up to date and very clearly written so as to avoid differing interpretation.

In health care institutions, job descriptions are based on the purpose, philosophy, and objectives of the nursing service department. They should be written so that the performance standards for any job can be identified. For example, if the nursing service department expects that all registered nurses will be responsible for ensuring that nursing care plans are up to date on the patients assigned to their care, then the job description should state, "Maintains current nursing care plans for all patients." It may seem that developing this degree of specificity about each position in an organization would be a never-ending job, but it actually saves time and misunderstanding once it is done. People understand what is to be done and who is to do it.

Understanding the Criteria for Evaluation

All employees should know the standards by which they will be evaluated. Evolving from job descriptions, these should be shared with the employee at the time of orientation to the job. Similarly, the purposes of evaluation need to be communicated and understood. The frequency of the formal evaluation interview also must be defined. In many instances, if the nurses operate within the guidelines of a negotiated contract with the hospital administration, the terms of evaluation will be described in the contract itself. Well-developed and implemented plans for monitoring the evaluation process and the tools used for appraising performance must also be in place. The accompanying display provides an example of "Guidelines for Performance Evaluation." These guidelines were incorporated into a contract between the Seattle Area Hospital Council and the Washington State Nurses Association, which negotiated the contract.

Guidelines for Performance Evaluation

Philosophy

An evaluation program should be considered as a step in bringing about, as well as determining progress in achieving personal and professional growth and development resulting in better patient care.

Principles and Guidelines

To meet evaluation criteria, a performance appraisal must be:

    a. Developed within the framework of the institution's written policies.
    b. Based on expectations as stated in the job description for the position.

(continued)

Guidelines for Performance Evaluation *(Continued)*

Philosophy

    c. Written and presented by an evaluator who has:
1. Been oriented to these Guidelines for Performance Evaluation and to the method of evaluation used in the particular institution.
2. Made actual and frequent observations of the performance of the evaluatee.
3. Been involved in the evaluatee's growth and development.

    d. Prepared prior to and presented in an evaluation conference which must be conducted by the person writing the evaluation. This conference must be conducted on a planned basis with foreknowledge of the evaluatee as to time and place.

    e. Prepared and presented prior to completion of the first ninety (90) days, no less than annually thereafter, and, if possible, at termination of employment.

    f. Presented with the understanding that:
1. The evaluatee has been oriented to these Guidelines for Performance Evaluation and to the method of evaluation used in the particular institution.
2. The evaluatee has the responsibility to participate in the evaluation conference by mutually planning, with the evaluator, personal and professional goals for further development.
3. The evaluatee may comment in writing on the evaluation form.

    g. Signed and dated by both the evaluator and the evaluatee to signify that the evaluation has been reviewed in conference.

    h. Reviewed, dated, and signed by a member of management in line authority above the evaluator.

    i. The nurse shall be given a copy of the reviewed, dated, and signed evaluation upon request.

    j. If a permanent nurse shall receive an evaluation that indicates unsatisfactory performance in some areas of practice, the nurse shall have a reasonable opportunity to improve, and then another evaluation shall be prepared and presented as above to indicate any change in performance, unless there is a clear and present danger to patients if the nurse remains in the nurse's regular assignment.

(Collective Bargaining Agreement by and Between the Washington State Nurses Association Northwest Local Unit and Northwest Hospital, July 1, 1985 to June 30, 1987.)

Knowing Who Will Be Evaluating Your Performance

All individuals employed in an organization must know who in that system is responsible for evaluating their performance. For example, you might be very distressed to learn that your evaluation was written by the day supervisor on your unit if you believed you would be evaluated by the charge nurse with whom you worked on the evening shift. In most organizations the employee will be evaluated by the immediate supervisor, because that person is most familiar with the employee's performance and the expectations of the position. Evaluations should be based on many different observations of performance, and the immediate supervisor usually works most closely with the subordinate.

However, the evaluation process may vary in certain institutions. If the immediate supervisor is not conducting the evaluation process, all efforts should be made to solicit accurate information about an employee's performance by the individual formally responsible for the process. It is also critical that the person doing the evaluating be skilled in conducting the appraisal interview and be trained in the use of the evaluation tool. In addition to an interview with the employee, the evaluation should be written and the employee should be given the opportunity to respond in writing. If the employee disagrees with statements in the evaluation, there should be a process for appeal. This highlights the importance of the employee knowing what is to be done with the written evaluation. Is it shared with the employee only? Is it shared with the employee and also placed in that person's personnel file? Is it transmitted to a person of higher authority in the organization?

A well-developed evaluation process is one that is viewed as fair and productive by all who participate in it and that has the support of top administration within the organization. These are also important characteristics of an effective system.

Types of Performance Evaluation Tools

A number of different types of evaluation tools exist. We shall not attempt to discuss all the forms in current use, but in the next few pages we shall share with you some of the more commonly used types of evaluation. It bears repeating that any evaluation must be based on frequent observations.

The Narrative or Essay Technique

In the narrative or essay technique the evaluator writes a paragraph or more (usually more) outlining an employee's strengths, weaknesses (or areas for improvement), and potential. It often begins with a brief description of the position the employee occupies within the organization and should always be reflective of the employee's performance in relation to the job description. It may also include some comment on personal attributes if pertinent to the job (*e.g.,* "ability to function well under stress"). This format for evaluation has the advantage of providing an in-depth review of an employee's performance and may be especially suitable for identifying problem areas and areas upon which to focus further development. However, its preparation can be quite time-consuming, can vary tremendously in length and content, and depends on the evaluator's ability to write. Narrative evaluations are difficult to compare, because each may touch on different aspects of performance. This form of evaluation is widely used in letters of recommendation.

Rating Scales

The rating scale is probably the most widely used comparison tool for evaluating nursing performance. The tool consists of a set of behaviors or characteristics to be rated (again based on the job description) and of some type of scale that will indicate the degree to which the person being evaluated demonstrates that behavior. The rating scale may take several forms.

Numerical rating scales. On numerical rating scales the degree to which the nurse meets a desired behavior is described by circling the appropriate number. Instructions on the evaluation instrument will state the levels; for example, using the numbers 1–5, the instructions will indicate that 5 is outstanding, 4 is above average, 3 is average, 2 is below average, and 1 is unsatisfactory.

Lettered rating scales. The lettered rating scales function in the same way as numerical scales except that letters are used instead of numbers. For example, outstanding performance may be represented by the letter *A;* above average, by the letter *B;* and so forth. One can quickly see how this could easily be equated with the "giving of grades" in our educational system.

Graphic rating scales. The graphic rating scale functions similarly to those just described except that the performance is rated by placing a mark somewhere along a horizontal line. The line is divided into sections with labels such as *always, frequently, usually, seldom,* and *never.* All standards of performance would then be listed on the evaluation tool and rated by this scale.

Descriptive graphic scales. Like the graphic rating scale, this form of evaluation tool describes in varying terms the degree of frequency with which the standard of performance is met, and these descriptions are placed along a continuum. For example, if the standard of performance relates to accurate and complete charting, the description at one end of the continuum might state, "Charts accurately and completely on all patients assigned, giving meaningful examples and observations." The statement at the opposite end of the continuum might state, "Charting is incomplete and not always accurate. Contains many misused and misspelled words." This would represent the best and worst behavior, and two or three additional statements describing other degrees of performance would be included along the line. As you have probably already determined, the development of this type of tool is very time-consuming.

Rating scales have the advantage of usually being very acceptable to the rater and providing information that is generally more consistent than that obtained in a narrative approach. However, it does not provide the depth of information that the narrative can make available, and its validity and reliability when used by different raters might be challenged. For example, what one head nurse may see as A performance may be rated as B performance by another head nurse.

The Checklist

Another type of evaluation form is the checklist. It describes the standard of performance and the rater indicates by placing a checkmark in a column if the staff nurse demonstrates that behavior. The columns are usually titled "yes, "no," or "not applicable," although other words carrying the same meaning can be used. These evaluation forms are efficient when evaluating a large number of employees but do not provide a way to indicate the degree or frequency with which a behavior occurs. Behavior is seldom either totally "yes" or totally "no."

Management by Objectives

During the 1960s, management by objectives gained a great deal of attention; as a result, evaluation tools were developed that incorporated this philosophy of management. They focus on the evaluator's observations of the employee's performance as measured against very specific, predetermined goals that have been jointly agreed upon by the employee and the evaluator. During the feedback interview the results are discussed and new goals for the next period of evaluation are established. This form of management and evaluation encourages employees' participation in setting their own goals and probably discourages their criticism that they are being judged unfairly. You can quickly imagine how this system would break down if the employee's goals differed from those of the organization or if the employee was not interested in establishing personal goals upon which to base evaluation. Management by objectives may not work in hospitals where the tasks (job description) of the nurse are based on patient needs that may vary and are therefore difficult to quantify and describe clearly.

Appraisal Methods Designed to Avoid Rater Bias

Several evaluation methods have the advantage of avoiding evaluator bias. Three such methods are the field review method, the forced-choice rating method, and the critical-incident technique.

The Field Review Method

The field review method allows the ratings of several supervisors to be compared for the same employee. A small group of raters is identified for each supervisory unit, and each rates an employee's performance. A member of the administrative staff then meets with the members of the rating group and identifies areas of interrater agreement. The administrative staff member helps the group arrive at consensus and helps each rater perceive the standards similarly. As you might anticipate, this can be very time-consuming.

The Forced-Choice Rating Method

The forced-choice rating method requires that the evaluator choose from among a group of statements those that "best describe" the individual being evaluated and those that "least describe" this person. The statements are then weighted or scored by another individual in the organization. High scores represent better employees. The evaluator does not know the scoring value of each statement while scoring, thus reducing bias. This method has the disadvantage of being costly to develop.

The Critical-Incident Technique

The critical-incident technique can be used in collecting data for application to some of the evaluation methods previously discussed (*e.g.*, the narrative method), or it can be used as a method itself. It requires that the supervisor observe, collect, and record instances of the employee carrying out responsibilities critical to the job. These are then used to prepare the evaluation or serve as the evaluation itself to be reviewed with the employee during the feedback interview. These written accounts of behavior tend to focus on performance rather than on personality traits and may assist the supervisors in their role as coach and communicator. Having to record incidents helps the supervisor remember more accurately and completely the aspects of an employee's performance for review at the time of the feedback interview. To be free of bias, it is important that incidents be recorded regularly and that they relate to job performance and job descriptions. The disadvantage of this is that it is time-consuming, because the supervisor must write down incidents on a regular basis. There is a tendency to record those behaviors that are not desirable and to fail to write down those that represent expected performance.

The Interview

Once the supervisor completes an employee's evaluation, time needs to be set aside to discuss the evaluation with that employee. This should not be the only time the supervisor communicates with the employee, but it can be one of the most meaningful. Certain characteristics can result in the interview being more successful.

Planning for the Interview

The review of an individual's performance should never be conducted haphazardly. The feedback interview may be more important to the entire performance evaluation system than the evaluation tools used to rate an employee's performance. A good interview requires thought and planning, just as other management activities do.

A specific, mutually convenient time should be set aside for the interview session. An interview conducted when the employee is concerned about completing the morning care of patients will not be as effective as one conducted when the employee can focus on the content of the interview. Similarly, an interview scheduled during a time when the supervisor is distracted by many other urgent items will result in hurrying through the process.

The interview should be conducted at a convenient, private location. A busy workroom or a corner of the nurses' station is not conducive to achieving performance review goals. It should be scheduled for a time that will allow for exchange of ideas and perceptions. It should not last longer than needed to accomplish specified activities; that is, it should not become the occasion for social chit-chat. Most interviews can be conducted in an hour or less.

Conducting the Interview

A good feedback interview allows both persons an opportunity to warm up for the session. Beginning with small talk will help the employee feel more at ease. Small talk about work-related situations tends to be more desirable than that about personal matters.

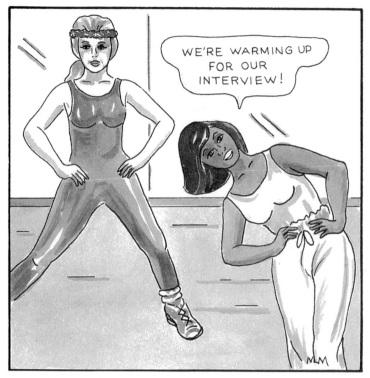

A good feedback interview allows both persons an opportunity to "warm up" for the session.

All information about performance provided to the employee should be job related and based on observed behavior. The ratings should be based on clearly defined expectations. There should be no surprises for the employee. Opportunity should be provided for an exchange of ideas and comments.

The manager should also anticipate that the employee may disagree with some of the comments made. The employee may have perceived his or her performance to be better than did the supervisor. Generally, open and candid responses are desirable in these situations, as is the ability to be a good listener.

Stevens (1975, p. 81) identified some common problems encountered in performance interview. These included the following:

- Conducting a one-way conversation
- Interrupting the employee's thoughts, explanations, or questions
- Criticizing the employee rather than the performance
- Smoothing over real deficiencies and problems too fast
- Failing to investigate facts before expressing opinions

- Passing the buck by claiming that one's corrective measures originate "higher up"
- Allowing the interview to fall into charge–countercharge styles
- Allowing the interview to fall into charge–excuse cycles
- Allowing the interview to deteriorate into a social visit

It is important that the nurse manager maintain control of the interview and ensure that productive communication patterns are used throughout. This can be encouraged if the nurse manager points out when a pattern or topic is not productive and redirects the conversation. It may also be useful to call the employee's attention to particular response patterns, such as excuses, that are nonproductive. Refocusing an interview is also a desirable way to maintain a positive discussion. Focusing evaluative statements on performance rather than on personality characteristics helps avoid areas that can disrupt the communication process (Haar, 1978).

When the evaluation conference results in a number of recommendations for change, it is desirable to arrange for a follow-up meeting. This will provide an opportunity for the employee to change his or her performance. In all instances it is important that the supervisor express confidence in the employee. The employee must understand that the manager believes the improvement will occur.

Responding to a Performance Evaluation

Much of this chapter has been written from the perspective of the beginning manager. However, as you begin your career in nursing you will be in the employee role rather than in that of manager. You will be participating in evaluation conferences as the follower rather than the leader. There are steps you can take in that role to ensure that the interview runs smoothly.

Certainly the guidelines outlined earlier with regard to informal feedback, both negative and positive, would apply to the formal evaluation process. In addition, in the formal evaluation process you may be asked to bring a self-evaluation to the interview or to respond in writing to a written evaluation that you will have discussed. If you truly disagree with comments that have been recorded, it is acceptable to make a written comment to that effect when signing the written document.

Most formal performance interviews are positive. The performance of an employee over the past 6 months or a year is reviewed against standards, goals may be set for the next period of time, and future plans may be discussed. If, however, the content of the interview is negative, you may find yourself feeling very defensive and perhaps emotionally upset. Continuing with the interview under these circumstances may not be desirable. It would then be appropriate to request that the interview be continued at a later time after you have had an opportunity to think about the comments that have been made. A second interview session could be scheduled in about 2 weeks. A statement such as, "I'm a little overwhelmed by the comments you have made. Could I have a little time to think about them before I respond—say, about 2 weeks?" would accomplish this.

PROGRESSIVE DISCIPLINE

There are times in any organization when the performance evaluation system must be used to determine whether an individual's employment should be terminated. The process of evaluating, providing feedback, and increasing sanctions on the employee is called progressive discipline. This occurs when, despite coaching and assistance, the employee's behavior continues to fall below the expected and allowable standard. This situation is taxing to the most experienced supervisor. Supervisors often dread disciplining employees. However, there will be times when patient safety or quality of care will demand it.

When the supervisor first realizes that there may be a serious problem requiring discipline, it is wise to contact the personnel department or the nursing director. Most contracts or policy manuals have sections that spell out the steps for dealing with instances in which the rights of the employee may be at risk (known as grievance procedures). It is important that persons to whom the supervisor reports are aware of the problem if it is going to require discipline. The situation should be discussed with them and approval obtained before moving ahead. The administration will want to be certain that the disciplinary steps are carried out fairly and are legally defensible.

Steps in Progressive Discipline

If progressive discipline becomes necessary, a series of steps should be followed. Needless to say, these start with the least severe and move to the more critical.

First of all, the employee must be counseled. When this takes place, the counseling should embrace all the guidelines discussed earlier as important to performance appraisal and negative feedback. Supervisors must have a good understanding of the strengths and limitations of their counseling skills. In most situations, matters discussed should be confined to those related to job expectations. Additional counseling of a personal nature might best be referred to a competent professional counselor.

The second step involves a reprimand to the employee and should be both written and oral. The employee must see and sign documentation that will verify that the problem has been discussed. Such documentation is usually placed in the employee's personnel file.

If the unacceptable behavior continues, the next progressive step is suspension. The employee will be told that he or she is not to return to work for a period of time—for instance, 3 weeks. It is hoped that this suspension will help the employee to see that the behaviors being exhibited are considered serious. Sometimes a suspension gives the employee the needed time to make some corrections.

When the behavior has not changed after the suspension, the final step is termination. In reality, many persons will terminate their employment voluntarily before reaching this stage in the process, but one cannot be certain this will always occur.

Critical Elements to Be Considered

Fortunately, most disciplinary situations can be handled informally. However, if the process becomes more formal, there are certain assurances that the supervisor must be able to make.

It is up to the employer to prove that the alleged acts did, in fact, occur and that they were sufficiently serious to warrant disciplinary action. (The ultimate in disciplinary action is often termination.) The burden of proof is placed upon the institution. When cases go to higher hearing boards, or perhaps into a court of law, the tendency is for a "poor little guy" attitude to prevail. It appears as though a large, profitable institution is against one little person who is trying to do his or her best. It is at times like these that the critical incidents or anecdotal notes compiled for the performance interview are so important. The records of all evaluations and evaluative sessions are also valuable.

The conduct that is being criticized must not have been condoned earlier. This means that it should not have been ignored or forgiven. Instead, the employee must have been specifically warned of the consequences of continuing the unacceptable behavior. Earlier in this chapter it was mentioned that some supervisors prefer to overlook poor performance rather than confront the employee. The importance of facing such problems head on is now more apparent. Think, for example, of the employee who you suspect of abusing alcohol or drugs. When unacceptable behavior is not dealt with openly, it is in reality being condoned. The employee is being given the message, "It's okay," or, "You're forgiven."

Most institutions have appeal boards or other processes for reviewing disciplinary cases. If these do not exist, individuals who believe they have been improperly treated may always seek retribution in our civil courts.

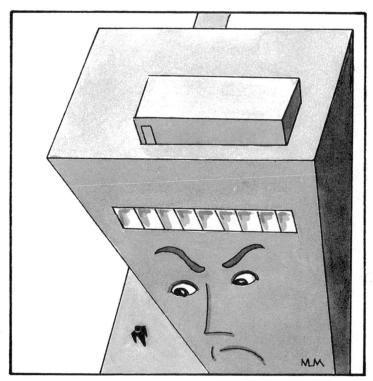

The burden of proof is placed upon the institution, for in hearings there is tendency for a "poor little guy" attitude to prevail.

To present a sound appearance if the process is challenged, certain elements are critical.

Proper and adequate documentation must be collected regarding the problems. This documentation must include a history of the incident(s). It is important that it not appear to be one person's word against another's.

In gathering the data for documentation, quick notes scrawled on a calendar or on a "daily reminder" will be useful. Most of us live busy lives, and it becomes difficult to recall exact times and dates if time has passed. The quick note should also include a short statement reminding you of the nature of the meeting, telephone call, message, or conference.

A written record of all conferences with the employee must be kept. These records must be shared with the employee, and in most instances opportunity must be provided for the employee to respond to them. When providing the employee with a copy of the record of the conference, it should be given in person. Leaving it in a mail box or some other place for "pick-up" provides no assurance that the employee will actually receive it.

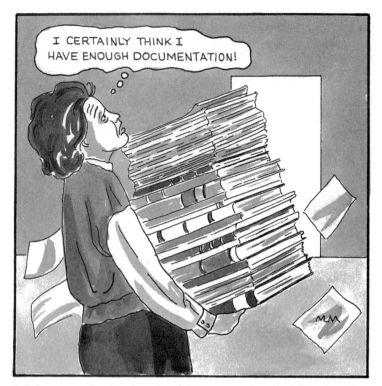

It is important in situations involving progressive discipline that adequate documentation be provided.

If it is anticipated that the conference with the employee will not go smoothly, it is desirable to have a third person present. The employee should know that this is to occur prior to the conference and may want to bring someone to represent his or her interests. If a contract is in effect in the organization, the employee's advocate may be a representative from the bargaining unit.

It must be clear to all that the employee has not been singled out for "disparate treatment." This means that other persons who perform the same acts must not have been excused. This may be one of the most difficult standards for a supervisor to maintain. For example, an employee who in other ways is an outstanding nurse cannot be allowed to be consistently late without reprimand if another individual is reprimanded for being late. Further, if a reprimand occurs it can only be for those behaviors that have occurred since the counseling session held earlier. For example, let us assume an employee is consistently late for work, is counseled, and improves. Then the employee starts making serious medication errors. The reprimand can deal only with the behavior related to failing to give medications correctly, because the previous problem has been corrected.

Information should be gathered that indicates that the misconduct was not of a temporary nature. We all have had "bad days" and sometimes "bad weeks." A consistent and recurrent pattern must be demonstrated that is unlikely to change in the future.

Guiding Questions to Consider

As with other areas of the appraisal system, progressive discipline has some common pitfalls. Some of these have been mentioned earlier but are again included so that you might see the total nature of the concerns:

1. Is there adequate documentation?
2. Has intervention occurred early enough?
3. Is there a job description and does the employee understand what is expected?
4. Does the employee know who will be doing the evaluation?
5. Has the supervisor erred in trying to be "too nice"?

Two other pitfalls of the progressive discipline system need to be discussed in more detail than a list allows. The first of these is the tendency to "overerupt" when "we've had it." Because managers are busy people, behavior that can be a serious problem is sometimes not addressed as early as it should be. There is a tendency to let it go until the manager can no longer tolerate it. Then the manager may overreact. This is a little like responding to a situation when one is angry, and it should be avoided.

The last problem is the tendency to write a glowing terminal evaluation for the employee when he or she leaves your employment. This evaluation could be used to discredit your previous statements if the matter were to go to a court of law. Informally, you may have to live with your words and evaluation if the person being evaluated seeks employment in a neighboring hospital or clinic. In either case, it is a situation to be avoided.

SUMMARY

Being able to provide and respond to feedback is a skill demanded of all managers. It requires that the individual be knowledgeable about both verbal and nonverbal behaviors and be able to use each effectively. Informal feedback involves providing the employee with day-to-day or hour-to-hour information regarding that employee's performance. This allows the employee to know if he or she is meeting the standards of the organization; reinforces good care, thus motivating the employee; and helps correct inappropriate or incorrect behaviors.

More formal feedback is known as performance evaluation. The most effective performance appraisal systems use evaluation tools that are built upon the employee's job description. The tools may take any one of several forms, including narratives, rating scales, checklists, management by objectives, or a method designed to avoid rater bias. Evaluations lead to a performance interview that should be well planned and conducted to allow for exchange of communication and feedback.

On occasion, the evaluation process must be used for assessing the need for progressive discipline and for carrying out the steps such action requires. The manager must be certain that he or she understands all the steps in the process and the common pitfalls encountered when implementing them.

Study Questions/Activities

1. What are the various parts of the communication process and why is each important?
2. What guidelines should be followed when communicating verbally?
3. What guidelines should be followed when communicating nonverbally?
4. What guidelines should be considered with regard to positive feedback?
5. How might you respond to positive feedback?
6. What guidelines should be considered with regard to negative feedback?
7. How might you respond to negative feedback?
8. What are the purposes of the formal appraisal from the point of view of both the employer and the employee?
9. What three characteristics are reflective of an effective performance appraisal system?
10. What are some of the various types of evaluation tools and what are the advantages and disadvantages of each?
11. Why is it important that evaluations avoid rater bias?
12. What are some factors that will result in the most successful interview?
13. How might one respond to a performance evaluation?
14. What is progressive discipline and when is it used?
15. What are the steps to be followed in progressive discipline?
16. What factors must be considered if progressive discipline is used?

17. What are some of the common problems associated with progressive discipline?

18. What are some of the questions that can be asked to guide a situation involving progressive discipline?

REFERENCES

Haar, L.P. (1978). Performance appraisal. In A.G. Rezler and B.J. Stevens (Eds.). *The nurse evaluator in education and service.* New York: McGraw-Hill.

Kron, T. (1981). *The management of patient care: Putting leadership skills to work* (5th ed.). Philadelphia: W.B. Saunders.

McGregor, D. (1972). An uneasy look at performance appraisal. *Harvard Business Review,* 44(5), 61–67.

Oberg, W. (1972). Make performance appraisal relevant. *Harvard Business Review,* 44(1), 62.

Stevens, B.J. (1975). *The nurse as executive.* Wakefield, Mass.: Contemporary Publishing.

SUGGESTIONS FOR FURTHER READING

Anderson, C. (1990). *Patient teaching and communicating in an information age.* Albany, N.Y.: Delmar Publishers.

Bushardt, S.C., & Fowler, A.R. (1988).Performance evaluation alternatives. *The Journal of Nursing Administration,* 18(10), 40–44.

Council, J.D., & Plachy, R.J. (1980). Performance appraisal is not enough. *The Journal of Nursing Administration,* 10(10), 22–30.

Drucker, P.F. (1974). *Management tasks, responsibilities, practices.* New York: Harper & Row.

Duldt, B.W., Griffin, K., & Patton, B.R. (1984). *Interpersonal communication in nursing.* Philadelphia: F.A. Davis.

Girard, R. (1988). Are performance appraisals passe? *Personnel Journal,* 67(8), 89–90.

Kjervik, D.K. (1984). Progressive discipline in nursing: Arbitrators' decisions. *Journal of Nursing Administration,* 14(4), 38–42.

Lachman, V.D. (1984). Increasing productivity through performance evaluation. *Journal of Nursing Administration,* 14(12), 7–14.

Levinson, H., & LaMonica, E. (1980). Ordinary M.B.O. appraisal process far from being a constructive technique raises great psychological issues. *Journal of Nursing Administration,* 10(9), 22–30.

Marriner, A. (1976). Evaluation of personnel. *Supervisor Nurse,* 7(5), 36–39.

O'Loughlin, E.L., & Kaulback, D. (1981). Peer review: A perspective for performance appraisal. *The Journal of Nursing Administration,* 11(9), 22–27.

Meeting and
Managing Conflict | 11

Objectives

After completing this chapter, you should be able to:

1. Discuss some of the early views of conflict.
2. Describe how conflict in organizations is viewed today.
3. List at least five positive outcomes of conflict.
4. Name at least four different contexts in which conflict occurs.
5. Identify and describe at least three causes of conflict.
6. Outline five modes or styles of dealing with conflict.
7. Describe a win–lose situation, a lose–lose situation, and a win–win situation.
8. List the steps to be considered in conflict resolution.
9. Discuss some guidelines to be followed in conflict resolution.

The topic of conflict will not be new to you. Conflict surrounds us and is a major concern of our human society. It is a part of everyday living. It has been with us since the beginning of time. Conflict between people keeps attorneys in business, supplies clients to marriage counselors, and challenges the most capable of parents to keep peace among children.

If you were raised in a fairly traditional family environment, you were probably taught that conflict was to be avoided, that peace and harmony were the desired behaviors. *Webster's New World Dictionary of the American Language* (1976) states that conflict refers to a sharp disagreement or collision in interest, or ideas, in which the process is more emphasized than the end. The word is derived from the Latin word *conflictus,* meaning "to strike together." Working from this definition, we shall think about conflict as a situation that exists when there is a difference of opinion or opposing points of view between persons, groups, or organizations.

EARLY VIEWS OF CONFLICT IN ORGANIZATIONS

As we examine literature in the area of management, we find that the early writers and theorists (called *traditionalists*) also held a negative view of conflict. They perceived conflict to be a disruptive and destructive force within any organization. The "good" manager was the individual who administered a unit free from conflict. In some early situations, the "troublesome" employee may have been dismissed from his job.

In the 1940s this view of conflict began to change. A new breed of theorists (identified as *behaviorists*) began recognizing the positive aspects of conflict. They recognized it for what it is—inevitable—and looked for ways to reduce it or to make it work positively for the organization. Some would say that this changing view of conflict, which occurred toward the end of World War II, was related to this country's involvement in nuclear strategies.

Organizational literature of the 1970s was replete with the examination, explanation, and positive application of conflict in the workplace. New theorists (called *interactionists*) emerged who viewed conflict as a creative force.

Assael (1969) described conflict as both beneficial and destructive. It is beneficial when it results in a more equitable allocation of political power or economic resources, but it is destructive when a lack of recognition of mutual objectives results. You can understand this concept better if you think of the conflict that can occur over the allocation of equipment or supplies to various areas within an organization. Suppose two different units are competing for money to buy equipment. A meeting is called and it is decided that both requests will be partially funded and that a request will be sent to the hospital foundation for the remainder of the funds. The conflict was viewed as beneficial. In the same situation, if a decision had been made to give the funds to one department and not to the other, or to give all the funds to yet another department, it would be seen as destructive, because there was a lack of recognition of mutual objectives.

PRESENT-DAY VIEWS OF CONFLICT

Today we tend to view conflict as inevitable and, if recognized and properly managed, capable of contributing positively to the operation of the organization. Lewis (1976) has described conflict as functional or dysfunctional (terms borrowed from organizational literature). Conflict may be viewed by some as functional but, at the same time, be perceived by others within the same organization as dysfunctional. For example, let us consider the decision made by a hospital to introduce a new system of patient care, moving from a team approach to one of case management. Staff nurses, who may not have been involved in the decision, might see the change as unnecessary restructuring requiring additional effort on their part. Some may see their role as threatened. This conflict could be seen as dysfunctional because it directed attention away from patient care.

The Positive Aspects of Conflict

Conflict within an organization can have many positive consequences. First of all, it often provides the impetus for change. A situation in which individuals or departments are struggling with one another must be resolved. Solutions must be found that will result in greater harmony. New methods, procedures, policies, or approaches will be searched for and implemented.

Conflict helps individuals understand one another's jobs and responsibilities. The more specialization that occurs, the greater the differences. The health care environment and the medical and nursing professions are becoming increasingly specialized. This provides a very fertile ground for conflict. In the process of looking for solutions to a problem, it is necessary to learn more about the other person and the factors that impinge on that individual's workday and responsibilities. This results in a greater appreciation for others on the team. Conflict situations provide an acceptable arena in which to bring differences in values and beliefs into the open, where they can be reevaluated or challenged.

Conflict may open new channels of communication. Meeting and settling conflicts involves defining and examining a problem. Both of these activities require skills in communication. In the process new approaches and avenues may evolve. In this sense, conflict can result in providing a formalized channel by which to express a grievance or one's dissatisfaction with the manner in which something is being done. In providing this pathway, accumulated hostility can be reduced.

Conflict serves to energize people. It wakes them up. One might wonder what there is in the nature of human beings that makes this true. Although we may not find an answer, we can benefit from the outcome. A spicy disagreement between departments or individuals tends to "get our attention" and adds a new dimension to the work environment. In this sense, conflict also provides an outlet for pent-up emotions. It provides an acceptable focus for expression of frustration. There are times in any organization when a staff group can be united by a threat or challenge from outside the group. An example might be a unit on which there has been a great deal of dissension among staff with regard to work schedules and provision of time off on weekends and holidays. A decision is made at a higher level in the organization to close the unit and relocate the

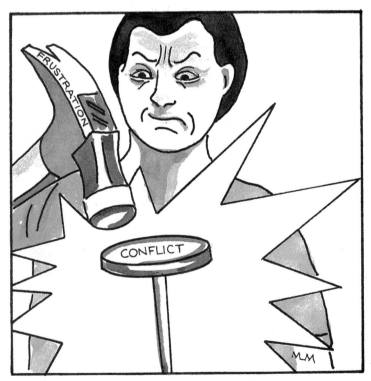

Conflict provides an outlet for pent-up emotions and an acceptable focus for the expression of frustration.

personnel in order to cut costs. Suddenly the individuals who were at odds with one another are pulling together to defeat the outside enemy.

Conflict may also result in a more equitable distribution of resources or power within an organization. Used in this sense, we are not limiting our definition of resources to strictly monetary ones; we also include responsibilities and roles and power within the organization (see Chap. 4 for a discussion of power). The process of defining the conflict brings concerns into the open, where positive alternatives are sought. Resolution may result in reallocation of money, time, or positions.

The Context in Which Conflict Occurs

Conflict has also been described and studied from the standpoint of where it occurs or of its context. One type can be described as intrapersonal, or occurring within the individual. Everyone is familiar with this type of conflict. You may recently have experienced it when you struggled with the decision of whether to study for an examination or watch your favorite television program. Conflict may be interpersonal. For example, you may have had a disagreement with a brother or sister during your adolescence about who would have the car on a given evening. Conflicts can occur among small groups, as one might see if two units were struggling over the use of a piece of equipment. Organization-wide conflict is also possible, as would occur, for example, if all the employees were up in arms about the salary and benefit plans being provided by the organization. And finally, conflict can occur between organizations or between the organization and its environment. A conflict over which one of two hospitals in a community should have a new oncology unit would be an example of this type of conflict.

TYPES AND CAUSES OF CONFLICT

Conflicts occur in our interpersonal relationships with others because of differing values, goals, actions, or perceptions. Similarly, conflicts occur in organizations because of differing perceptions or goals. Marriner (1979) defines these conflicts as being either horizontal or vertical. Horizontal conflicts are those among individuals who occupy equal or similar positions within an organization (*i.e.,* they appear on the same level on an organizational chart) and have to do with authority, expertise, and areas of practice. Vertical conflicts involve lack of understanding between superiors and followers, as would be seen in differences in perception of role, poor communications, or incompatibility of expectations. The identification of superior–subordinate conflict has led to the development of modes of resolution, to be discussed later in this chapter.

One of the areas responsible for much conflict is that of role conflict or ambiguity. Role conflict occurs when there is uncertainty about the work expectations related to unclear or inadequate information. This would include situations in which there is a blurring of roles or role competition. Two persons have related responsibilities and it is unclear where the boundaries are. For example, in some hospitals there has been a conflict between the nurses on the unit and the social work department about the responsibility for providing discharge planning. Both areas saw it as an important aspect of their care of the patient. Another example of role conflict and blurring of responsibility occurs when a person's position in the organization requires him or her to wear a number of hats, such as the night supervisor who must be a skilled care giver, a teacher, a negotiator, a patient advocate, a manager, and a motivator. The requirements of one position may be in conflict with those of another. As you can easily surmise, the individual experiences role conflict and much stress; consequently, productivity and job satisfaction are reduced. This type of role conflict is a major cause of burnout.

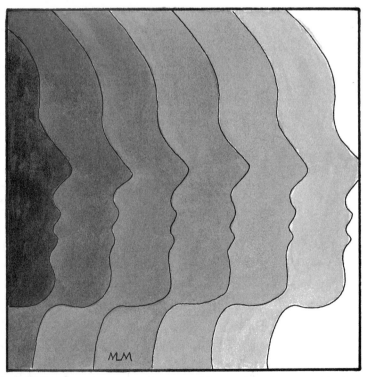

Conflict can occur in situations where there is blurring or ambiguity of roles.

The structure of the organization may be another source of conflict. To minimize this we use job descriptions, organizational charts, and other such mechanisms. This type of conflict increases as organizations increase in size. The less control individuals have in planning their work, the greater the conflict. For example, think of the nurse who cannot begin the patient's morning care until the patient has had breakfast. The patient cannot have breakfast until she has had a fasting blood sugar drawn. The personnel from the laboratory are delayed in coming to the unit because one of the technicians called in ill and no replacement could be found. All persons in this conflict feel the stress of the situation. This type of conflict is most apt to occur within an organization when units depend on one another for assistance, information, and other types of coordination.

Conflict also results from a scarcity of resources. As mentioned earlier, this is not limited to monetary resources; it may also involve personnel, positions, space, or other elements critical to the operation of any unit within an institution. For example, the size and location of one's office or the number of people required to share an office or a telephone line are very common sources of conflict within organizations and may relate to an individual's perceived power within the group.

RESOLVING CONFLICT

Given the inevitability of conflict and the fact that it can have positive outcomes within an organization, resulting in growth and improved relationships, we are challenged to find the most effective ways of resolving it. Certainly the approach that one would use depends upon the nature of the conflict, the characteristics of the individuals involved, and the personal skills of the individual responsible for seeing that a resolution occurs. Some persons are intimidated by conflict. Others are all too ready to "take on the world." Just as planning care for your patients requires a thorough assessment of all related factors, which you have already learned, so does conflict resolution.

A wide variety of approaches to the management of conflict exist. Although some may be more desirable, when viewed in total perspective, than others, any one of them may be useful in selected situations. A wise manager selects the approach that best fits the situation. This selection is based on the relative importance of the issue, the potential for positive outcomes, and the energy and time available.

Several researchers interested in learning more about conflict believe that individuals possess behavioral predispositions or personal styles for handling and resolving conflict (Berkowitz, 1962; Thomas, 1962; Blake & Mouton, 1964). These styles tend to fall into one of five different categories.

Avoiding or Withdrawing from Conflict

Avoiding or withdrawing from conflict is generally seen in individuals who are made very uncomfortable by conflict situations. This may also be referred to as denying conflict. Those who employ this tactic often do not see any positive attributes in conflict. They tend to cope well in situations in which there is harmony but will not become involved in conflict. Think for a minute. Do you know someone who fits this description? Perhaps you are such a person. Do you prefer to remain neutral when a conflict occurs, avoiding situations that might require you to take sides? Although avoiding conflict may result in less upset, it may also result in the organization losing important information. Each of us brings special skills, abilities, and perceptions to a work environment. These should be shared in bad times as well as good times.

> *Example:* You are in the line in the hospital cafeteria and have only 20 minutes for your lunch. The area is very busy. The clinical nurse specialist who has been visiting your mastectomy patients prior to discharge crowds in front of you in the salad line. Rather than challenging her boldness, you just step back. You have had a particularly hectic morning and, in addition, you are counting on a recommendation from this individual for a merit increase.

Smoothing, Suppressing, or Accommodating to Conflict

Persons who usually choose to smooth, suppress, or accommodate to conflict situations are often described as having a strong need to be liked and are concerned for the welfare and needs of others. If a conflict situation threatens how they will be perceived by others or presents too many challenges to someone important to them, they try to accommodate to the problems. In striving to maintain a peaceful environment, personal goals and values must be sacrificed. Accommodators can fill a positive role in a conflict situation by providing support to others involved in making tough decisions. However, in accommodating to the situation the individual may be abandoning responsibility for providing valuable input to problem resolution. Have you been in conflict situations where you wanted to share information that you had but where the cost of friendship or discomfort with others stopped you? Most students can think of a time during their schooling when they were aware of cheating or plagiarism by a classmate and struggled with the decision of what to do. Similar conflicts will follow you into the work environment. Do you report a colleague that you know is taking supplies from the unit? Is it more serious if you know an individual is charting assessments he or she has not done? How will you handle these situations?

Example: You walk into the utility room and find one of the new staff nurses in tears. When you ask what is bothering her, she states, "Dr. Bellows just chewed me out because I didn't have size 8½ gloves available for him." You have been meaning to talk with Dr. Bellows about the manner in which he treats new employees; however, he has just been made Chief of Staff. You put your arm around the new employee and say, "Dr. Bellows likes to eat new staff for breakfast. Now you are initiated! He'll leave you alone next month."

Compromising or Negotiating Conflict Situations

The approach to conflict that employs compromise or negotiation of conflict situations is one of give and take. One factor in the situation is balanced against another. This method of conflict resolution works because it minimizes the losses for all parties while providing some gains. The difficulty with an approach that involves compromise is that the problem often resurfaces. In deciding to use compromise to resolve a conflict, you need to assure yourself that this is the best way to deal with the situation and that it is not just the easy way out. You have used compromise throughout your life to deal with conflict. Perhaps when you were growing up you negotiated with a brother or sister regarding duties ("I'll mow the lawn if you'll rake the leaves," or, "I'll do the vacuuming if you will do the dusting"). In such situations compromise helped accomplish the task and the approach did not warrant any more consideration than it was given. In other situations, however, more thought should be given to the solution of the problem.

Example: You are meeting with two other unit managers regarding the budget for next year. Each of you needs several pieces of relatively expensive equipment. Your unit really needs a machine that would take the entire budget allocation. Rather than push for the most expensive piece, you suggest that if each of the others will reconsider their requests, you will delay a year in asking for the more expensive item. This approach would allow each unit to purchase some of the items they need.

Forcing the Issue or Competing

Persons who address conflict in a competitive manner emphasize personal goals and desires and fail to consider the needs and opinions of others. These individuals have a strong need to come out of any conflict situation as "the winner." Although this aggressive approach may serve to move issues that are deadlocked, it can prevent good problem solving. The competitors win by out-talking their colleagues, by discounting the good ideas presented by others, or by personally attacking others. You can all think of an example of a conflict that was resolved with the use of the competitive approach. It may have involved something as simple as deciding with a friend whether you would eat at one restaurant or another.

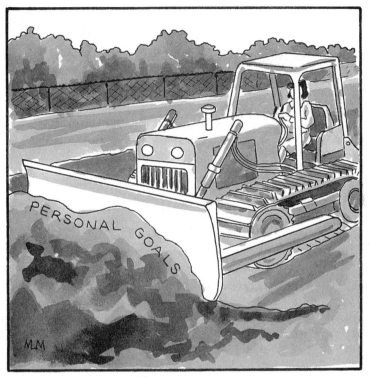

Some persons address conflict in a competitive nature, pushing personal goals and desires.

You will want to develop the ability to know when a competitive approach to a problem is desirable and when another method should be employed.

> *Example:* At a meeting of the procedure committee the technique to be used in cleaning a tracheostomy is being reviewed. Although you know that several approaches are correct, you have just read a new article researching this topic. It is important to you that you influence the decision and that the new technique be adopted. You know that the reading you do and your verbal skills will intimidate others into accommodating to your position. Therefore, you talk at some length about the findings of the research. The technique you are proposing is adopted.

Problem Solving or Collaborating

Many studies of conflict resolution advocate a problem-solving or collaborative approach while acknowledging that it may be the most difficult to achieve. This method encourages the individuals involved in the conflict to work toward common goals. However, it requires that all persons come to the discussion table willing to examine issues thoughtfully and work in a task-oriented fashion to solve the problem. It requires a commitment on the part of all persons to be supportive and considerate of one another, to listen to the other person, and to try to understand that person's point of view. It demands awareness and sensitivity. It would, for example, break down if one of the individuals was approaching the problem from a competitive stance.

> *Example:* You are working on a unit where different nurses are assigned to various management activities. The one for which you are responsible is the scheduling of hours. Much dissension occurs on the unit with regard to the scheduling of weekends off. You decide to call all unit staff together to discuss the problem and establish the criteria by which weekends off will be rotated among staff. The goal is to involve everyone in the decision making.

Personal Styles and Conflict Resolution

In addition to the techniques just described, each of us brings to the conflict situation our own patterns of response. Some of these are helpful in terms of resolving a conflict; others not. The manner in which we respond to a conflict situation is determined by the degree to which we are willing to assert ourselves in the attempt to achieve our goals and aspirations and the degree to which we are willing to assist other in accomplishing their goals and desires. Filley and Kerr (1976) have developed a table that identifies three basic personal styles, which they have named *Tough Battler, Friendly Helper,* and *Problem Solver.* Table 11-1 helps you to anticipate the outcome when these various types come into conflict. Review this table and consider how you fit within the descriptions. What role do you most often see nurses adopting? What skills will be needed to assure greater success in a conflict situation?

TABLE 11-1. OUTCOMES IN COMBINATIONS OF PERSONAL STYLES IN CONFLICT NEGOTIATION

	Tough Battler	Friendly Helper	Problem Solver
Tough Battler	Stalemate 80%	Battler wins 90%	Battler wins over 50%
Friendly Helper	X	Stalemate 80%	Problem solver wins
Problem Solver	X	X	Quick agreement

(Filley, A., House, R., & Kerr, S. [1976]. *Managerial process and organizational behavior.* Glenview, Ill.: Scott Foresman and Co.)

OUTCOMES OF CONFLICT

In looking at the outcome of conflict, Filley (1975) has identified three different positions. You have heard these terms used in your everyday experiences with others.

The *win–lose* outcome occurs when one person dominates the situation and the other individual submits. Often the domination occurs because of power or authority within the organization or situation. A win–lose outcome can also result from mental or physical coercion. Of the styles described in the preceding section, forcing, competing, and negotiating would most likely result in win–lose outcomes. This type of outcome may have positive benefits in certain circumstances. There are occasions when it may be the only appropriate approach (*e.g.,* if you find yourself in disagreement with your supervisor about the details to be reported on an incident report and about the depth to which they should be described). There may be little to be achieved by making this a major issue, and your supervisor's authoritative position will provide leverage within the organization. However, if the same persons or groups are consistently on the losing end, productivity and cohesiveness will be diminished, and eventually leadership will be challenged. On occasion, solutions are referred to as win–lose/win–lose. This means that each participant won some and each lost some.

In the *lose–lose* situation there are no winners; the resolution of the conflict is unsatisfactory to both parties. Of the styles discussed earlier, smoothing and compromising would fall into this category and so, on occasion, would avoiding and withdrawing. The most typical example of this situation can be found in the arena of labor negotiations. When the contract negotiation process stalemates and goes to arbitration, a third person is called in to mediate or decide the outcome. The result may be one that involves sufficient compromise to render it unsatisfactory to both sides.

Win–win outcomes are, of course, the most desirable. In these situations, both parties walk away from the conflict having achieved all or most of their goals or desires. The problem-solving or collaborating style discussed earlier most often leads to win–win situations.

Let us look for a minute at some of the characteristics of these various outcomes and relate them to everyday occurrences. When we are working with individuals in groups, there is a common tendency to decide issues by *majority vote*. Certainly that is how our political leaders are selected and how motions are decided in formal meetings. Somebody (or one group) wins and somebody (or one group) loses. In these situations that is the most orderly way in which to conduct the activities. However, when trying to achieve common goals for a unit or department, working toward *consensus* (agreement among group members) may provide for greater harmony in the long run. Consensus building may appear to take more time, and obviously requires interpersonal skills on the part of the leader, but it results in easier implementation, because of group acceptance. This avoids some of the "we–they" positions taken in both the win–lose and the lose–lose strategies. It allows both sides to look at the conflict as a problem needing resolution, tends to depersonalize the issues, and emphasizes outcomes.

There are times in a conflict situation when the needs or desires of the involved individuals or groups become polarized. That means they are diametrically opposed or at opposite ends of a continuum. In these instances focusing on the means to resolving the problem rather than on the outcomes may be desirable. This approach is known as *integrative decision making*. The persons involved spend time identifying their needs and values, search for all possible alternatives, and then select that which works best. This method tends to bring attention to the problem rather than to the persons involved.

Groups are affected by winning. Winning tends to increase cohesiveness among members and to create a more relaxed climate in which to function. Concern for the members' needs increases, and at the same time, concern for task performance or orientation declines.

Similarly, groups are affected by losing. There is a tendency to deny the reality of losing, excusing it as the result of bad luck or misunderstanding. Internal conflicts may occur as members blame one another for the defeat; there is a tendency to work harder and to reorganize in order to be more effective.

THE STEPS IN CONFLICT RESOLUTION

As you approach a conflict situation with the goal of seeking an equitable resolution, there are a series of steps you will want to follow. The first of these involves self-assessment. If you are going to attempt to resolve a conflict, you need to ask yourself first if you have a complete understanding of the problem. What factors may limit your understanding? Is your perception of the situation accurate? Where can or should you go for more information? Are there factors in the conflict that bias you one way or another? Are there alternatives to solving the problem that are clearly to be avoided? Do you have the resources, either personal or material, to resolve the conflict? Is the conflict one that should be resolved? Are we hearing what we really think we are hearing? What will be the harm to the organization if it is not resolved? Conducting this type of assessment may deescalate the problem.

Next you will want to conduct an analysis or review of the issues and conditions surrounding the conflict. In conducting this type of review, you might discover that the problems can be easily resolved by adjusting a condition that led to the conflict. For example, there was conflict among nurses on a particular unit in the hospital because the time allowed for all employees to take a 15-minute morning coffee break extended from 9:15 to 10:00. This was an insufficient period of time to allow all employees a 15-minute break. Employees began to challenge one another over who could go first, second, third, and so forth, with the last group often not having time for a break. Much energy was being invested in trying to remember or track who had had the first break the day before, and the day before that. By analyzing and reviewing the situation rather than the conflict itself, it was easily solved by adjusting the time allowed for the coffee break. An additional time period was added, and some employees were permitted to take their 15-minute break a some point between 8:15 and 8:45.

The third step involves reviewing and adjusting attitudes. If you find, for example, that you have certain biases regarding a person or situation, those biases must be adjusted before beginning to resolve the conflict. Our attitudes provide the screen or sieve through which we receive and give information. They can serve to distort or warp data being provided to us. It is important that we be able to discriminate between situations in which we are dealing with facts and those in which we are dealing with feelings and to put each in the proper perspective.

Having completed these initial steps in the assessment, we are ready to move on to more tangible aspects of conflict resolution. You will recognize these as similar to the steps of the nursing process that you learned early in your nursing studies. These represent the steps in integrative decision making or problem solving discussed earlier.

The persons involved in the conflict are called together to work on the problem. People should be notified in advance of the meeting, the time, the place, and the issue to be discussed. Although this may initially create some anxiety among participants, advance notice tends to lessen the emotional impact and eliminates the discomfort individuals experience in surprise meetings for which they cannot psychologically or mentally prepare. This results in greater trust being established. The meeting should occur on "neutral" ground and privacy should be assured. Sufficient time should be allotted to permit full discussion of the issue.

During the meeting each individual should be encouraged to express his or her views, perceptions, needs, and goals. A climate must be created that will encourage and support a free exchange of ideas and attitudes. This step in the resolution of the conflict will result in the identification of the problem. It is important that the problems be fully defined before solutions are outlined. There are times when the full magnitude of the conflict is not brought out because of personal tensions or the desire to get things over with as quickly as possible. It is important to continue active questioning until all issues are identified. All participants should be encouraged to share both positive and negative thoughts. It is important that the person responsible for providing leadership to the group be able to discourage behaviors that are destructive to this process. All points of view should be accepted and all perceptions taken seriously.

With this completed, we are ready to move on to developing and outlining solutions. At this point in a conflict situation there is a psychological lift in the process. Individuals feel relieved to have gotten through the problem. It is important to look at all the alternatives to solving the problem, even those that may seem to have little relevance, merit, or impact on the situation. All persons should be encouraged to supply solutions to the problem. Just as they are involved in the conflict, they must also be involved in finding the solution. At this point in the resolution process, it may be appropriate to seek outside help or information. Use of outside resources is common in integrative problem solving.

Identification of solutions concludes with a narrowing of choices for action. Criteria for evaluating the merit of the various alternatives must be established. Different approaches to the problem should be discussed and the best solution identified. Again, all persons must be involved in this process, for this results in a commitment on the part of all individuals to see that it is implemented or carried forward. If some members in the group need to change their behavior, this is most apt to occur if they have exercised an instrumental role in identifying the solution. If solutions are suggested that some members of the group cannot support, discussion should continue until alternative methods are identified.

Before attempting to implement the solution or activities it necessitates, you should clearly understand and communicate who is to do what and in what time frame. A written plan for implementation or an implementation table may be useful, a copy of which can be shared with all. This plan or table should also deal with the time lines. During this process criteria for evaluating the outcome should be defined. Persons need to know how they will monitor the process and how they will assess whether it is working. This helps to build in accountability and ownership for seeing successful completion of the plan.

GUIDELINES FOR DEALING WITH A CONFLICT SITUATION

Conflict situations can be exhausting and time-consuming. It is useful to review some basic guidelines for dealing with conflict situations before jumping head first into the problem. You will recognize many of these guidelines as similar to those described in Chapter 10 (Providing Feedback and Evaluation). You will also recognize that many of these are basic to positive interpersonal relationships, but it is often the interpersonal relationships that suffer in a conflict.

First of all, you want to deal with the issue, not the personality. By focusing on the problem at hand and not the characteristics of the persons involved, each party is able to maintain his or her self-respect and self-esteem.

Give positive feedback when good ideas are presented. Keep the discussion open and the atmosphere accepting. It is more important that all views be heard than it is to have a peaceful meeting.

Give all persons an equal opportunity to be heard and assure that their statements are listened to actively. In one meeting in which some participants had a tendency to do more than their share of talking and occasionally tried to talk at the same time, the leader distributed poker chips. Blue chips were worth 5 minutes time, red were worth 3, and white were worth 1. Chips were distributed equally to all participants, who bought time by throwing a chip to the center of the table. This helped to lend some degree of order to the discussion and encouraged all participants to think about what they were going to say before using up their time.

Clarify positions presented by others by restating them or rephrasing them. When the listener rephrases a statement, it provides assurance that it was heard as intended. In the feedback loop this would be similar to correct decoding of the message by the receiver.

If the discussion promises to be a hot one, establish game rules before beginning. Be certain that all participants understand what behavior is acceptable during the session and what is not. Once rules have been established, be certain that they are followed. Let us say, for example, that it is decided that dehumanizing behaviors such as laughing at the way an individual describes feelings or putting down that expression by verbally discrediting it will not be allowed. If halfway through the discussion one member says to another, "I can't imagine why you would feel that way!" it is important for the leader to stop the discussion and remind participants of the rules.

SUMMARY

Conflict occurs when individuals, groups, or organizations hold differing values, goals, or perceptions. Conflict is inevitable in our society and can have positive outcomes if managed appropriately. Conflict can provide an impetus for change, can help individuals understand one another's jobs and responsibilities, opens new channels of communication, energizes people, and may result in a more equitable distribution of resources within an organization.

Conflict can occur within the individual, between individuals or groups, or between organizations or the organization and the environment.

Conflict occurs because of blurring of roles or role conflict, the structure of the organization, or scarcity of resources with the organization.

When managing conflict several different styles may be employed. These include avoiding or withdrawing from the conflict; smoothing, suppressing, or accommodating to the conflict situation; compromising or negotiating around the conflict situation; forcing the issue or competing; and problem solving or collaborating. Problem solving may represent the best approach to conflict and may also be the most difficult to achieve.

The outcomes of conflict resolution can be viewed as creating a win–lose situation, a lose–lose situation, or a win–win situation. Win–win situations most often result when an integrative decision-making approach is employed.

Before attempting to resolve conflicts, you should assess yourself and your attitudes, assess the issues or conditions surrounding the conflict, and review and adjust your attitudes. The steps to conflict resolution are similar to those you learned in the nursing process and include gathering data about the problem, defining the problem, outlining all alternatives, identifying and implementing the best alternative, and evaluating the outcome.

Interpersonal skills in managing conflicts include dealing with the situation not the personality, providing all persons with equal opportunity to present their views, clarifying statements, and establishing and enforcing ground rules.

Study Questions

Situational Questions

At 8:00 A.M. Mary Jones, the head nurse on the medical unit, calls the hospital laboratory area to question why a blood sugar has not been drawn on one of the patients on her unit. As she slams down the phone she states, "I get so exasperated waiting for those lab people to get their work done! They think they are the only ones in this organization that ever run short-staffed. I'm going to talk to someone about this."

1. What is the source of this conflict?
2. In which context does this conflict occur?
3. If you were Mary's supervisor and responsible for seeing this situation resolved, where would you begin? Why?

4. What style of conflict management would you choose? Why?

5. What would be your reasons for not choosing one of the other styles for managing this conflict?

6. What might be some of the positive outcomes of this conflict?

You walk into the utility room and find the staff nurse and the ostomy nurse in a heated argument over who should be teaching the patient care of his colostomy.

7. What is the source of this conflict?

8. What steps might be taken to prevent it from happening in the future?

9. How would you deal with the situation in the utility room? Why did you choose that approach?

General Questions

10. How do early views of conflict differ from present-day ones?

11. Why is majority vote considered a win–lose situation?

12. Why is consensus building a desirable method to use in conflict resolution?

13. Why does employing a labor mediator in a negotiation stalemate run the risk of resulting in a lose–lose situation?

14. What steps should be followed in resolving conflicts?

15. Of the guidelines for resolving conflict provided in this chapter, which do you believe is most important? Why?

REFERENCES

Assael, H. (1969). Constructive role of interorganizational conflict. *Administrative Science Quarterly, 14*(4), 573–582.

Berkowitz, L. (1962). *Aggression: A social analysis.* New York: McGraw-Hill.

Blake, R., & Mouton, J. (1964). *The managerial grid.* Houston: Gulf.

Filley, A. (1975). *Interpersonal conflict resolution.* Glenview, Illinois: Scott, Foresman & Co.

Filley, A., House, R., & Kerr, S. (1976). *Managerial Process and Organizational Behavior.* Glenview, Illinois: Scott, Foresman & Co.

Lewis, J. (1976). Conflict management. *Journal of Nursing Administration, 6*(10), 18–22.

Marriner, A. (1979). Conflict theory: Its sources, its uses. *Supervisor Nurse, 10*(10), 12–16.

Thomas, K. (1976). Conflict and conflict management. In M. Dunnette (Ed.), *The handbook of industrial and organizational psychology.* Chicago: Rand McNally.

Webster's New World Dictionary of the American Language, 2nd College Edition. (1976). D.B. Guralnik (Ed.). Cleveland: William Collins + World Publishing.

SUGGESTIONS FOR FURTHER READING

Ambrose, J. (1989). Your power to resolve conflict in the professional setting. *Today's OR Nurse, 11*(3), 13–21, 30–32.

Edmunds, M. (1979). Conflict. *Nurse Practitioner, 4*(4), 42, 47–48.

Isaac, S. (1986). Five ways to resolve conflict. *Nursing 86, 16*(3), 89.

Loraine, K. (1989). Winning strategies when the game is confrontation. *RN, 52*(3), 18, 20.

Mallory, G. (1985). Turn conflict into cooperation. *Nursing 85, 15*(3), 81–83.

Marriner, A. (1982). Managing conflict. *Nursing Management, 13*(6), 6.

Todd, S. (1989). Coping with conflict. *Nursing 89, 19*(10), 100, 102, 105.

Becoming an Effective Advocate   12

Objectives

After completing this chapter, you should be able to:

1. *Recognize several definitions of advocacy.*
2. *Identify concepts related to advocacy.*
3. *Discuss reasons for being an advocate.*
4. *List goals of patient advocacy.*
5. *Explain behaviors that exhibit patient advocacy.*
6. *Recognize effective strategies for patient advocacy.*
7. *Discuss supports and constraints of the advocacy role.*

HISTORICAL BACKGROUND

Traditionally in our society, the sick role has granted persons two privileges and required two obligations. The privileges include being released from normal obligations, such as work, and being the recipient of appropriate care. In return, the ill individual should make every effort to seek help and to comply with the advice given to achieve recovery (Parsons, 1951). This view places the patient in a very dependent, unquestioning role. The only responsibility for one's own health is the responsibility to carry out the health care provider's instructions or to be compliant with the physician's plan of care. This view supported and perpetuated the paternalistic health care system (Webb & Merritt, 1989). *Paternalism* is the restricting of an individual's liberty by making decisions for the person, in the manner of a father making decisions for his children. It usually involves withholding information and is justified because the decision maker "knows what is best" for the person. Traditionally, citizens credited the physician with knowing what was best, did not seek information, and allowed the physician to make choices for them.

In the 1960s and 1970s the complexity of the health care system increased. Many highly technical machines and chemical treatments were developed, greatly increasing the alternatives and consequences of decision making. Public knowledge of the treatment protocols and their consequences was limited. Inadequacies, as well as capabilities, of our health care system were publicized more widely. Consumers in general demanded increased status and power. Defenders of patients' rights proliferated and challenged the paternalistic health care system. Patients began to demand their right to make health care decisions and to receive the information necessary to make those choices. The distance narrowed between the consumer and the provider of health care. There was increased emphasis on consumer needs and rights in all areas of health care.

Several documents reflected the changing view of the patient's role, rights, and responsibilities. The American Hospital Association Patient Bill of Rights was written. A Nursing Home Patient Bill of Rights was developed. The American Nurses' Association Code of Ethics was changed to give specific support to advocacy of patient rights. The American Association of Colleges of Nursing published the seven values essential for a professional nurse, which included the necessity of honoring the individual's right to refuse treatment and the obligation of the nurse to act as a health care advocate.

In 1978 federal legislation required each state to set up an ombudsman program for nursing homes. Hospitals began to explore the need for a salaried position of patient advocate, separate from all of the service departments in the agency. The governmental concept of representation entered the health care field.

For nursing, advocacy is rooted in the values for dignity and freedom of the individual client and in the importance of client education. The advocacy role evolved as the nursing profession became increasingly autonomous and client centered. Initially, the advocate role involved being an actor for or on behalf of another. Then the nurse advocate acted as a mediator between the client and other persons. Finally, the nurse became a protector of clients' self-determination (Nelson, 1988). The progression of the role has increasingly involved the client in decision making and self-care.

DEFINITIONS

Definitions parallel the three-stage historical development of the concept of advocacy. Alfano (1987) puts two of Webster's definitions together to define *patient advocate*. An advocate is one who pleads another's cause, especially before a judicial court. A patient is defined as a person awaiting or receiving medical care, receiving personal services, and/or being acted upon. Therefore, a patient advocate is one who pleads the cause for those receiving medical care or personal services before those who could deprive them of such services. Other authors concur. Kosik (1972) defines an advocate as one who intercedes for another or for a group of people.

Bernhard and Walsh (1981) say advocacy is supporting, defending, and maintaining the cause of someone or something. Van Kempen (1979) writes that an advocate is one who defends or intervenes on behalf of another and who acts for, and in the interest of, the client's welfare.

The second definition addresses *mediation*. It states that an advocate defends a cause or speaks and writes in support of a particular belief or program. The purpose of mediation is to arrive at a solution that is acceptable to all persons involved: those making the decision and those affected by it. This aspect of advocacy can include political action to influence public policy relevant to health.

Currently, the most prevalent definition emphasizes the importance of individual rights and self-determination. Advocacy is defined as helping patients to be autonomous, informed decision makers. The best interests of the patient are determined primarily by the patient, not by nurses or other professionals. This definition requires that nurses and patients interact as whole and unique persons to determine the meaning of the experience for the client. Giving advice is no longer sufficient. Teaching and support are given according to client needs and choices. This moves advocacy from interceding or pleading a case for the client to actively promoting the client's rights to autonomy and free choice.

Zussman (1982) identifies two types of advocacy roles. One is the *responsible* model, which utilizes negotiation, compromise, and persuasion. It involves interaction with other persons associated with the situation. The second type is the *adversarial,* or legalistic, model. In this model the advocate acts as an adversary to other health care professionals without regard to the rights of anyone except the patient.

A patient advocate differs from a consumer advocate, who provides information then withdraws and allows the person to make a decision. A patient advocate differs from a patient representative, or patient rights advocate, who is employed by the facility and is available to deal with all patient complaints after they are made known. A patient advocate differs from an ombudsman, who handles grievances to protect the resident's confidentiality and rights. A patient advocate is not a rescuer who usurps the client's responsibility and rights, nor is the advocate paternalistic, making decisions about what is best for others based on his or her own principles and values and then forcing the beneficiary to accept the decision for his own good. A patient advocate is one who, depending on the situation, speaks for the patient, mediates between the patient and other persons, and/or protects the patient's right to self-determination. Areas of study that are important to, but different from, advocacy are ethical issues, legal issues, social issues, and political issues.

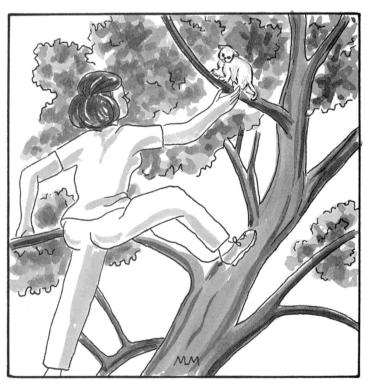

A patient advocate is not a rescuer.

REASONS TO ADVOCATE

Reasons for advocacy exist because, in our complex health care system, a client may be unable to verbalize needs or desires, may disagree with powerful others, or may lack the knowledge and support to make and implement health-related decisions. The following are broad goals for advocacy:

- To ensure that patients, family, and health care professionals are partners, especially when treatment is long, involved, and costly
- To involve citizens in the decisions that affect their lives
- To leave power with the patient while giving information, counsel, and services
- To help patients cope with complex physical, psychological, financial, and social problems
- To safeguard the interests and values of individual patients
- To provide a better quality of life
- To provide knowledge, understanding, and suggestions of alternatives
- To add humaneness to acute medical settings
- To increase palliation for terminally ill persons
- To increase respectful behavior toward patients
- To promote acceptance of patient choice, even when that choice is refusal of treatment or medications
- To help patients do what they deliberately choose to do
- To prevent denial of patient rights.

REASONS FOR NURSES TO BE PATIENT ADVOCATES

Nurses function as patient advocates to meet patient needs and to meet their own needs. Whereas ombudsmen and patient rights advocates intervene only if a problem is identified, nurses can be intermediaries for *all* persons who enter the maze of the health care delivery system.

Compared with other health care professionals, nurses spend more time in contact with patients and provide intimate physical and emotional care. This allows better understanding of patient needs and values and promotes trust relationships. Nurses are with patients when crisis or distress is immediate and decision making is essential. Nurses can use their understanding of patient needs and values to provide guidance in decision making.

Nurses are available to speak for clients, and daily interaction with other health care professionals is part of the nursing role. Communications can be expanded to incorporate advocacy and increase the nurse's feelings of power, adequacy, and achievement.

Nurses are very knowledgeable about the patient as a human being and are concerned about quality of life and death. Being an advocate is part of providing care that is morally and ethically right. Being an advocate is part of functioning as an effective leader.

PREREQUISITES

Before being a patient advocate, you must identify and define your own beliefs and values. What do you believe about advocacy (positive and negative outcomes, constraints and supports), patient roles and rights, professional behavior, and patient–family–physician relationships? Which do you value more: safety or freedom, obedience or questioning, compliance or autonomy? Are you willing to take calculated risks, initiate interdisciplinary communications, address problems considering multiple alternatives? How important to you are comfort, dignity, peace, control, knowledge? Who receives your loyalty—the physician, hospital, patient, or all three? Who is in charge of the client's well-being? Do patients have the right of self-determination? Are you willing to give up your authority and control over the client?

An adequate educational and experiential background is necessary before advocacy can be accomplished. Do you have knowledge of and experience in problem solving, values clarification, negotiation, mediation, and assertiveness? Can you assess each patient, including the level of autonomy desired and the ability to function outside the protected and structured hospital environment?

Adequate education and experience produce clinical competence, which is necessary to achieve the patient trust and respect that are prerequisite to advocacy. Clinical competence gives you greater credibility with colleagues and increases your success as an advocate. Understanding of the health care system, good working relationships, and communication with other health care professionals are all part of competent clinical practice.

To be an advocate you must believe that you have the right to speak up. Advocacy requires a decision to view yourself in a particular way in your relationship to others (Epstein, 1982; Kohnke, 1982). You must accept accountability for exercising the privilege and responsibility of advocacy. You need to consider how you will interact with persons who elect not to make a decision or elect to allow powerful others to make decisions for them. How will you advocate for the silent patient? Can your actions be justified, because patient self-determination requires rational thought and standard communication (Gadow, 1989)?

Close contact with the patient and patient trust are prerequisite to patient advocacy. You need skills that go beyond informing and supporting and that include helping the client to examine and prioritize values, recognize conflicts, and consider consequences adequately. Before you speak for a person or group, be sure that you represent their values, views, desires, and decisions and not your own.

Your personal attributes can influence your ability to serve as a patient advocate. Helpful personal attributes that facilitate advocacy are self-motivation, objectivity, empathy, tact, flexibility, tenacity, a sense of humor, ability to cope with stress and pressure, personal commitment to the patient, power, and personal autonomy.

CATEGORIES OF RECIPIENTS

Persons who can benefit from advocacy are those who lack knowledge or power, who are undecided about ethical dilemmas, and who receive inadequate care. Knowledge deficits may relate to patient rights, rules of the health care system, prognosis, treatment options, and available resources. At-risk clients include those who are participating in research and those who are terminally or chronically ill.

Persons who are attributed less power are those who are unconscious, silent, poor, young, old, or mentally ill. Ethical decisions relate to many interventions: restraints, feeding tubes, ventilators, institutionalization, specific medication, and so forth. Sometimes advocacy is needed to assist the client to decide. Sometimes it is needed because the client has not been given the option to make decisions.

Persons who receive inadequate, unsafe, or indifferent care may take their case to various advocacy groups or persons, but nursing always has a responsibility to address, secure, and ensure quality patient care.

SPECIFIC OBJECTIVES OF ADVOCACY

Broad goals toward which the nurse should strive are listed earlier in the chapter as reasons to advocate. Specific objectives related to feelings, knowledge, and behaviors of the patient are included here. The patient will

- Understand the rights of patients and be afforded those rights.
- Be informed about the diagnoses, treatment, prognosis, and choices.
- Have increased autonomy, power, and self-determination.
- Have decreased anxiety, frustration, and anger.
- Receive humane and just treatment and equality of opportunity.

- Take responsibility for his or her own life, so that decisions can be made in collaboration with others.
- No longer be threatened by those who know best.
- Have continuity of care and effective, efficient resolution of specific problems of care.

NURSING ACTIONS TO ACHIEVE THE GOALS OF ADVOCACY

To achieve patient advocacy, nurses may be required to interact with many persons, individually or in groups. Those most often involved are family members, physicians, and other health care personnel. Others include neighbors, employers, state agencies, and third-party payors.

Specific nursing interventions relevant to advocacy fall into the following seven categories:

1. Preventing the need for advocacy
2. Assessing the need for advocacy
3. Communicating with other professionals
4. Providing information and education to the patient
5. Assisting and supporting the patient's own decision making
6. Working for needed changes in the health care system
7. Being involved in public policy formulation.

Intervening to Prevent the Need

All nurses can assist the patient and physician to gain the best possible control over the disease manifestations that interfere with thinking, feeling, and doing. We can help prevent the need for advocacy by insisting on clear, agreed-upon health care goals and treatment strategies developed by a team that includes the patient or patient representative. We can be clinically competent, maintaining excellence in all aspects of patient care. We can be knowledgeable about cultural values and practices of individual patients and communicate these to other health care personnel while emphasizing that excellent care means individualized care. We can assist the patient to find and arrange appropriate and competent services as they are needed. You should be able to cite many examples from your own experience of situations in which advocacy was unnecessary. These might include situations in which the patient remained alert, capable of thinking and problem solving.

> *Example:* All health care personnel who interacted with the patient considered his individual needs and desires, provided him information, and involved him in decisions. The patient involved the family as he chose. The patient's progress was as expected, and needed services were available and arranged before discharge.

Assessing the Need for Advocacy

Your assessment of the need for advocacy should include the patient, the situation, the options and resources, the post-hospital setting, and the risks. This section will focus on patient assessment.

It is important for you to know the role the patient chooses, the role of significant others in health care decisions, and the role the nurse is expected to play (Becker, 1986). Does the patient expect to make his own decisions? Does he expect his wife or son to make needed decisions? Will he accept all decisions made by the doctor? Does he want the nurse to provide guidance in decision making?

You should be aware of the patient's concerns, questions, desires, and expectations. Consider the spiritual needs because they influence the beliefs and values that underlie the patient's decision making (Salladay & McDonnell, 1989).

It is important to assess the patient's desire to know. Miller's (1981) research showed that some patients cope better with little information about threatening events whereas others cope better with much information.

> *Example:* Mrs. Bateen is 79 years old and was admitted for removal of a tumor from the colon. Her husband has always made decisions for the family after discussing things with her. She has "faith in the doctor to do what is right and will do, pretty much, whatever he says." She does not ask questions but listens to instructions and explanations about her illness, hospitalization, and health-related behaviors.
>
> Based on this assessment, you anticipate all essential questions that she "should" ask (based on your knowledge and questions that other patients in similar situations have asked) and share the answers to them in a concise, understandable manner. You provide the teaching when her husband is present and ask him if he has questions. You ask the physician to reinforce essential instructions. You discuss discharge needs and plans with Mr. Bateen and confirm with Mrs. Bateen that they are appropriate and acceptable.
>
> Although you may want to assist Mrs. Bateen to be assertive and independent, you must consider her values and desires and, after acknowledging your own, set your own aside and work within hers.

Communicating with Health Care Professionals

It is important to communicate clearly with nurses and other health team members. Establish trust between yourself and other health care personnel. To do this you must demonstrate knowledge, tact, and a balance of objectivity and subjectivity. Communications with other professionals will include the rights and needs of patients as well as the patient's concerns, questions, and expectations. You can assist others in remembering and honoring patient rights and in showing respect. A team approach is facilitated by making other professionals aware of information that you have shared or are planning to share with clients and family members. Although speaking for patients is one definition of advocacy, it is best to encourage communication between the patient and health care providers. Speak for patients only when they cannot or are afraid to speak for themselves.

When calling physicians about patient problems or requests, call the appropriate physician. For example, call the surgeon if the problem is related to the incision or the system that was operated on. Call the internist if the problem is related to preexisting conditions treated by the internist, complications of immobility, or other nonsurgical complications affecting the heart, lungs, peripheral circulation, and so on. When requesting specific orders, particularly related to services after discharge or alternate care options, seek out the appropriate physician who is most responsive to these areas of need. When requesting or discussing plans for alternative care, present a knowledgeable, logical, concise, convincing argument.

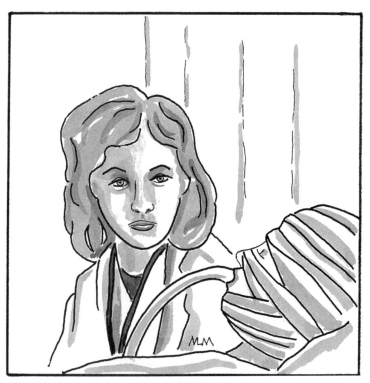

An advocate speaks for a patient only when he is unable to speak for himself.

When you are the manager, be sure that scheduled appointments are made in a rational way to prevent long waits in radiology, clinics, offices, and admissions. Coordinate services with the patient's time, energy, and needs in mind. Articulate roles and relationships between and among health care providers so that the patient is not caught in the middle.

Physicians and administrators need to be maintained as allies. To achieve this, you should state disagreements clearly, choosing wisely the time, place, and persons involved. Problems must be presented to appropriate colleagues with possible consequences and solutions. Negotiation and compromise are used to resolve conflicting interests between patient and provider. You can work with ombudsmen and other advocacy persons and groups.

> *Example:* Mrs. Childers is 48 years old and was admitted for a mastectomy. The cancer has metastasized to the bone. She has always made her own decisions, and her husband is very supportive of her and of her decisions. They are intelligent and have ample financial resources but very little knowledge of the health care delivery system, illness, possible treatment alternatives, and their expected outcomes. Mrs. Childers says the physicians plan to do a radical mastectomy, followed as soon as possible with intensive inpatient chemotherapy. She would prefer a modified radical mastectomy and "a little time after I recover from the surgery to have quality time with my family and do a few things that are very important to me before I get sick from the chemo." She has many questions about hospital routines and expectations, about her rights as a patient, and about options and prognosis.

After validating your assessment, you would plan for intervention. Write, and begin immediate implementation of, a teaching plan covering all her questions and concerns. Involve nursing staff on all shifts. If there are questions that you believe other health team members could answer better than the nursing team, call the appropriate department to share the question or concern and ascertain the answer or schedule a meeting with Mrs. Childers and the health team person. Include Mr. Childers if he and she both want him to be there.

Before you discuss the treatment options with the physicians, ask Mrs. Childers how she wants the situation to be handled: Does she want to initiate the conversation with them after you explain her rights? Does she want you to bring up the issue when both you and the doctor are in her room? Does she want you to speak for her and talk with the surgeon and oncologist about both the surgery and chemotherapy when she is not present? This will require your willingness and ability to function as a protector of patient self-determination, as a mediator, or as one who speaks for another.

It is best to handle this as a team player and not as an adversary. Negotiation and compromise may be necessary if the physician insists that the chemotherapy will be much more effective if it is started as soon as it can safely be administered. The compromise will include medications and other interventions to control undesired side-effects and planning quality time based on expected control of the side-effects.

> *Example:* In an 11 P.M. report, the nurse stated that Mrs. Spencer, a 72-year-old woman admitted on the day shift, had pulled out her NG tube more than once on evenings. She was alert and oriented to person, place, and time. She stated she did not want the tube and had resisted its repeated insertion. The staff had applied restraints to facilitate tube insertion and maintenance. Her children wanted it in. They did not believe she was capable of making her own decisions. The doctor had ordered the tube insertion and tube feeding. The tube was out at the change of shift.
>
> Ronda Tirey, the night charge nurse, did a Mini Mental Status assessment when she made first rounds. She talked with Mrs. Spencer about her health, the need for the feedings, and the reasons for removal of the tube. Mrs. Spencer's score indicated that she was mentally competent. She was also able to take oral fluids.
>
> As the nurse left the room, Mrs. Spencer's primary physician was standing at the nursing station. The patient's behavior, mental status, and rationale for refusal were presented to the physician. Ronda also stated that, because the patient had a right to refuse, the feedings and restraints were inappropriate (as well as ineffective); she would not reinsert the tube. She added that the doctor could do it if she still believed it should be in place, or another nurse in the institution would probably do it.
>
> The physician indicated that she had ordered it because the children had insisted and she had not had enough data to justify a denial, even though she had questioned the need. She expressed appreciation for Ronda's assessments and decision and used them to support her own decision. She ordered the tube discontinued and arranged for continued independent living for Mrs. Spencer on her discharge.

Providing Information and Education

Many patients need help to interpret hospital policies, health problems, procedures, services, and their own rights so they can make informed choices. In your nursing courses and clinical experience, you have acquired knowledge that you can share with patients. Education is the central activity of advocacy. The first step in communicating with and educating patients is to establish trust between yourself and each patient. Being honest and avoiding false reassurances are helpful in establishing trust. Resist the temptation to say, "Everything will be fine," or, "You'll have to stay here until you get better," when you know the patient will not get better.

You must possess the necessary knowledge and the communication skills to convey that knowledge. Then you can answer patient questions honestly and correct misconceptions that are expressed. Increasing your own knowledge base may make it more difficult to use appropriate terms that the patient can understand, so guard your word choice as well as the accuracy of the information that you share. How you say something is as important as what you say. Your attitude and intonation should convey caring and encourage further information-seeking or clarification.

Knowledge about current trends and about the legal and ethical implications of giving information is vital to the nurse who educates clients. Consider the source of the information, who should provide the information and be responsible for its use, and when and how it is to be given.

Allow the patient to select the information that will be received but do not wait to be asked for information. Encourage each patient to seek information from multiple sources and enable selection of the information that is meaningful. It is appropriate for you to include your own views. State them as your views and do not present them from a position of power or as a persuasive or coercive force (Corcoran, 1988).

It may be necessary to teach assertiveness so a patient can feel and act like an equal partner in communication, decision making, and treatment (Palmer & Deck, 1987). This requires special knowledge and perhaps an extended time period with the patient. Role playing can allow the learner to practice assertiveness.

Because children experience higher levels of anxiety and fear when they are uncertain about care procedures and what they can expect or

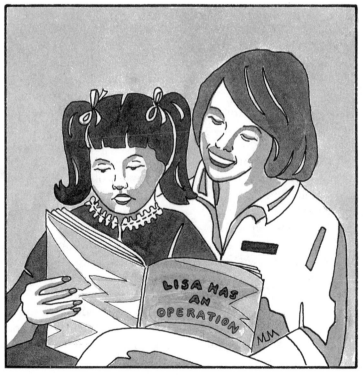

Because children experience higher levels of anxiety, they should be included in the information-sharing experience.

anticipate, they should be included in the information-sharing experience. Use content and approaches learned in your pediatrics course.

Family members are partners in the education process. They need information about alternative care, especially when they must choose interventions that would be acceptable to and in the best interests of a relative who is unable to make his or her own decision. If appropriate, you can remind them of the patient's expressed or written wishes.

> *Example:* Mr. Mathis is 24 years old and has just been diagnosed as having type I diabetes mellitus. He lives alone and does his own cooking except when he goes home, when "Mom expects me to eat everything she prepares and is insulted if I don't." He exercises regularly. He graduated from high school but does not like to read and does not read well.
>
> The obvious teaching relates to the multiple areas of diabetic instruction, planning for the use of nonwritten material when possible. Advocacy may be needed with employer and/or third-party payors to arrange for the client's participation in a diabetic teaching center program.
>
> The less obvious advocacy role may involve advocating with the mother or assisting the client to advocate for himself related to meals at the mother's home. This probably will necessitate assisting the mother to identify the significance to her of "eating everything" and to find other ways to meet her need for feeling needed and appreciated.

Assisting and Supporting Client Decision Making

You can help your patients to identify their own (not yours, not a significant other's) values and to decide accordingly. Assist your patient to prioritize values and to consider conflicts and consequences of choices. Help him or her to move through the steps of problem solving to become clear about the chosen behavior. Being sensitive to patient needs and experiences increases trust in you and makes you more understanding and effective in facilitating problem solving.

You can assist your patient to find meaning in illness as well as to reach decisions about the management of the illness. When appropriate, help the patient and family come to terms with imminent death (Epstein, 1982; Salladay & McDonnell, 1989).

For decision making, individuals need to know options available, chance events associated with each option, the probabilities that the chance events will occur, outcomes that may result, and their own values assigned to the outcomes (Corcoran, 1988). This gives further credence to the need for client education, as presented in the previous section. Including the physician, other care providers, and the family in discussion of the preceding aspects adds to the information shared and to the acceptance of the information.

A caring atmosphere is enhanced by showing respect for each patient and by supporting individual decisions, even if you disagree with the choices. You may need to set aside personal preferences and utilize unit politics to make it possible for patients to set and achieve goals.

You empower persons by giving them control. You can allow and encourage a patient to practice the assertiveness that was discussed in the previous section. As part of assertiveness, you can assist individual patients to present deliberative choices to other persons involved in the decision-making process. You can help the patient to formulate thoughts, questions, statements, and decisions and even rehearse conversations that will be used to present their views to others.

> *Example:* After many months of chemotherapy, Mrs. Childers is readmitted with complications of treatment and increased symptoms related to the cancer. She recognizes you and asks you to plan time to talk with her. You know this session will require more than providing information to a patient and are not sure about your readiness to interact on a more difficult level. Yet you understand the need for Mrs. Childers to identify her values related to the illness, to define the meaning of her illness and possibly of her death, and to make decisions about how and where she wants her future treatment or refusal of it implemented. You may need to advocate for in-home hospice instead of hospitalization. This advocacy may be with family or physician.

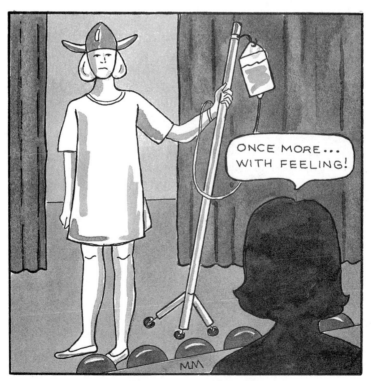

You can help patients rehearse conversations that will be used to present their views to others.

This situation requires not only using therapeutic communication techniques but also conveying caring and support to Mrs. Childers. It may require that you tolerate your own discomfort in order to listen to concerns, decisions, and acceptance or lack of acceptance of the prognosis. Do you remember "therapeutic use of self" from your psychiatric course? This is the time to use it! It is also time to use values clarification and problem-solving techniques in an interpersonal environment of caring. If you have not learned these skills, practice and perhaps continuing education workshops are appropriate.

Working for Changes in the Health Care System

Another path for advocacy is working for change in the health care system. You must know the bureaucracy in which you function. Find out about the powerful committees and meet the nurse representatives who serve on them (Nelson, 1988). It is always appropriate to challenge incorrect or ineffective policies and procedures and to work to change them. Advocate a policy; propose a policy; oppose a policy. Help define code status and other ethical issues. Volunteer to be on or work to establish an ethics committee in your institution.

The practice of nurses collaborating with and supporting other nurses in multiple professional activities has increased greatly throughout the past few years. Your collaboration with and support of nurses who are functioning as advocates is another part of your own advocacy.

Resources should be available so that patients can select options that fit their values and choices. If a needed service or facility does not exist, assist in its creation. Clearly state the patients' needs. Know how much needed services will cost and how much it will cost not to have the service. When community services do exist, they should be well organized, so that persons can know what is available, where it is available, to whom it is available, and how to gain access.

Your goal is to assist in making changes without making enemies. Use assertiveness with tact and planned strategy. State expected outcomes specifically. Be sure that your behavior is consistent with your expressed values underlying the request for change. Collaborate with the responsible persons in each situation using established channels of communication that provide the highest probability of success.

Working to prevent or correct incompetent, unethical, or illegal practice by any health care provider is part of professional practice. Sometimes advocacy is necessary to deal with situations involving unacceptable practices.

Example: Community Hospital did not have a written policy about significant others being in the room during a code situation; however, they were always kept out of the room. Jeanna Brooks, ER charge nurse, had talked with nurses who worked in hospitals where a significant other was allowed to be in the room during a code. The interactions and results sounded promising. When she asked about the practice at Community, she was told, "It has always been that way and it is best that way." She read and made copies of articles that pertained to the topic. She presented her position, with references, to her immediate supervisor and was given time to meet with the Policy and Procedure Committee. Using the hospital policy format, she wrote a draft of her proposed policy and took it to the committee meeting. She also provided names of ER nurses (with their permission) who worked in ERs that had implemented similar policies.

Being Involved in Public Policy Formulation

As a citizen, each of us has the privilege and obligation to be actively involved in government and in the policies formulated by our elected and appointed governmental personnel. You can become politically competent first as a citizen then as a health care professional. Contact your congressional representatives in support of legislation that benefits patients or makes needed services available to them. Offer to serve on health policy task forces and committees. Be actively involved in nursing organizations that work for programs and services for patients and network through professional organizations, alumni groups, friends, and co-workers.

Example: Jeremy Zinc had worked with in-home elderly for 3 years. He knew that several of his previous clients could have remained at home if the home health agency had offered, through their own department or by referral, part-time daily companion services. He had worked with a local task force to create the service, but the administrative expenses involved made the service too expensive to implement. Knowing that the State Nurses' Association was concerned about this need and was planning to approach legislators about introducing a bill to address the need, he asked to be involved with the district and state legislative committees of the association. He worked with a subcommittee to prepare a comparison of the cost of this program with the cost of institutionalization. He actively recruited other nurses and concerned persons to interact with their legislators in support of the bill to create the needed service as an expansion of the state health program.

CONSTRAINTS

Constraints to advocacy exist in many forms. Some of the hindrances are presented in this section.

There can be conflict of interest for the nurse between interests of an individual patient and the duty to serve other patients, self, the profession, and/or the institution. Often there is a lack of support for the advocacy role from institutions or other professionals.

Nurses may feel that they do not have the necessary knowledge or judgment to advocate. They may perceive a greater obligation to the employing institution and the physician than loyalty to the client. Advocacy may be viewed as bucking the system, thus creating undesirable risks for the advocate. There is the risk of being caught in the middle when all involved believe they know what is right for the patient. Based on knowledge and/or previous experience, nurses may fear legal or social consequences of advocacy and find it more appealing to do only what is ordered. The experience of Jolene Tuma discouraged many nurses from functioning in an advocacy role.

Jolene Tuma shared information about alternatives to cancer chemotherapy. The physician sued for interference with the doctor–patient relationship. Tuma lost her job and license to practice nursing. The license was later reinstated (Tuma, 1977). It would have been easier and less threatening if she had not intervened. Would the patient's quality of life have been as good? (Perhaps a less disruptive strategy would have included the patient's family and physician in the discussion of options presented to the patient.)

Nurses may believe that being a team player and presenting a unified, competent team image is more effective in building patient trust and confidence, and therefore more desirable, than is advocacy. They may concur with a perceived public view that the physician is the sole authority and decision maker in health care situations or perceive themselves as lacking authority and power.

Patients who have control and practice self-determination may be threatening to individual nurses. There may be fear of noncompliant patients who ask too many questions. Nurses may disagree with the decision made by the patient and not want to assist in the implementation of the decision.

Advocacy requires time, energy, flexibility, cooperation, and giving up power to the patient. It can increase the conflict with other health care personnel, who may not want to share their knowledge or authority.

SUPPORTS

The major support for the advocacy role is the reward the nurse receives from knowing that patients are receiving quality care in accord with their rights and without sacrificing their dignity. The personal growth of clients, in participating in goal setting and achievement and in accepting responsibility for the consequences of care, adds to the nurse's reward and encourages future advocacy.

If advocacy is approached in a professional manner, collegial communication and cooperation are improved. Positive interdisciplinary experiences increase feelings of self-worth and contribute to a pride of team accomplishment.

With the advent of consumerism, feminism, and the shift in power to the health consumer, the risks for the patient advocate are decreased. The advocacy position is strengthened by the increasing support for the belief that the interests of both health care providers and health care consumers are best served by effective consumer participation at the decision-making level. The legal mandate for informed consent supports the educational activities relevant to advocacy.

ADVOCATING FOR STAFF MEMBERS

Staff members, as well as patients, may benefit from the advocacy of a nursing manager. The first-line manager frequently represents the staff in meetings with other departments and upper management. Managers must speak to staff needs, requests, problems, and rights. A sensitive, effective leader consistently advocates for his or her group and for individual staff members whenever the need arises.

> *Example:* You are the evening charge nurse on the skilled unit of a nursing home. As report is concluded, your regular aide, Tina Hall, enters the conference room. She is obviously upset but only asks about her assignment for the evening. When you ask if she wants to discuss whatever the problem is, she states that the director of nursing just chewed her out because she was late. Because of her home situation, she sometimes has to ride with another person and cannot control precisely the time of her arrival. You know that she is an excellent, efficient, and caring aide. She does her share of the evening work and performs better than many of the employees.
>
> You know that lateness must be discouraged. However, because of your concern for the well-being of your residents and your concern for your staff person, you talk with the director of nursing. You state your assessment of the situation, emphasizing the importance of retaining Tina and supporting her decision to work even when it is difficult for her to make the necessary arrangements to do so. You suggest that she should be commended for her quality patient care and that mutually acceptable ways should be negotiated to compensate for her lateness when it occurs.

SUMMARY

This chapter has presented the history and definitions of advocacy, reasons to advocate, prerequisites of the art, goals and recipients of advocacy, and concepts related to the role. Based on the historical development and present status of the concept, the three definitions of advocacy involve speaking for or on behalf of the client, mediating between the client and another person, and protecting the client's self-determination. The primary goal of advocacy is to ensure patient rights by providing information and power as needed by the patient to increase feelings of control, respect, humaneness, and partnership. Prerequisites to advocacy are the belief that it is appropriate, and at times essential, to effective nursing care and the knowledge and skills necessary for the achievement of successful advocacy. Ethical, legal, social, and political issues are areas of study that are related to advocacy.

Emphasis has been on nursing actions to achieve the goals of advocacy, with the goal that patient, and perhaps staff, advocacy will be an integral component of your chosen role—that you will continually add to your knowledge and practice of advocacy as you add to your knowledge and practice of new technologies. Specific nursing interventions relevant to advocacy include (1) preventing the need for advocacy, (2) assessing the need for advocacy, (3) communicating with other professionals, (4) providing information and education to the patient, (5) assisting and supporting the patient's own decision making, (6) working for needed changes in the health care system, and (7) being involved in public policy formulation.

Constraints and supports for the role must be considered before you choose to be an active advocate. Will advocacy enhance or prejudice your relationship with patients, their significant others, the employing agency, physicians, and/or other nurses? Do the potential benefits outweigh the risks? Only you can define your role, examine patient rights and your duty, establish your priorities, evaluate the risks, and resolve inner conflict so that you can function effectively as an advocate at the level you choose.

Study Questions/Activities

1. Should nurses be advocates? Do nurses have the power, knowledge, and interpersonal skills to be advocates?
2. Copy each goal of advocacy on a separate sheet of paper. Under each goal list all the nursing actions that facilitate its achievement.
3. Study each example in the chapter. For each one identify for whom the nurse is advocating (*e.g.*, patient, family member, staff person), with whom the nurse is advocating (*e.g.*, physician, administrator, nurse, family member), establish a goal of the advocacy process for that situation, and state the definition of advocacy that applies.

4. Again look at the examples given. Discuss possible constraints to advocacy specific to each one. What negative consequences could occur for the nurse? For the client?
5. With other classmates, discuss situations from you own clinical experiences when you or a staff nurse advocated successfully or unsuccessfully. What knowledge or strategies differed in the two situations? What behaviors demonstrated patient advocacy?
6. Identify two categories of recipients for which there is no example given. Write your own example.

REFERENCES

Alfano, G.J. (1987). The nurse as patient advocate (editorial). *Geriatric Nursing, 8*(3), 119.

Becker, P.H. (1986). Advocacy in nursing: Perils and possibilities. *Holistic Nursing Practice, 1*(1), 54–63.

Bernhard, L.A., & Walsh, M. (1981). *Leadership: The key to the professionalization of nursing.* New York: McGraw-Hill.

Corcoran, S. (1988). Toward operationalizing an advocacy role. *Journal of Professional Nursing, 4,* 242–248.

Epstein, C. (1982). *The nurse leader: Philosophy and practice.* Reston, Va.: Reston.

Gadow, S. (1989). Clinical subjectivity: Advocacy with silent patients. *Nursing Clinics of North American, 24,* 535–541.

Kohnke, M.F. (1982). *Advocacy: Risk and reality.* St. Louis: C.V. Mosby.

Kosik, S.H. (1972). Patient advocacy or fighting the system. *American Journal of Nursing, 72,* 694–698.

Miller, S. (1981). Predictability and human stress: Toward a clarification of evidence and theory. *Advanced Experiments in Social Psychology, 14,* 203–255.

Nelson, M.L. (1988). Advocacy in nursing. *Nursing Outlook, 36,* 136–141.

Palmer, M.E., & Deck, E.S. (1987). Teaching your patients to assert their rights. *American Journal of Nursing, 87,* 650–654.

Parsons, T. (1951). *The social system.* New York: The Free Press.

Salladay, S.A., & McDonnell, M.M. (1989). Spiritual care, ethical choices, and patient advocacy. *Nursing Clinics of North America, 24,* 543–549.

Tuma, J. (1977). Letter to the editor: Professional misconduct. *Nursing Outlook, 25,* 546.

Van Kempen, S. (1979). The nurse as client advocate. In C.C. Clark & C.A. Shea (Eds.), *Management in nursing: A vital link in the health care system* (pp. 184–197). New York: McGraw-Hill.

Webb, E., & Merritt, J. (1989). Rights and wrongs. *Nursing Times, 85*(7), 59.

Zussman, J. (1982). Think twice about becoming a patient advocate. *Nursing Life, 6,* 46–50.

SUGGESTIONS FOR FURTHER READING

Anderson, D. (1989). Advocacy for AIDS patients is helping all patients. *RN, 52*(2), 65–72.

Backus, L.V., & Inlander, C.B. (1986). Consumer rights in health care. *Nursing Economics, 4,* 314–317.

Beaman, J. (1989). Patient advocacy: Should I or shouldn't I? *Imprint, 36,* 155, 157.

Barrett, J.E. (1987). In search of advocacy. *American Journal of Nursing, 87,* 1730.

Bujoran, G.A. (1988). Clinical trials: Patient issues in the decision-making process. *Oncology Nursing Forum, 15,* 779–783.

Copp, L.A. (1986). The nurse as advocate for vulnerable persons. *Journal of Advanced Nursing, 11,* 255–262.

Evers, L. (1987). AIDS and confidentiality. *AD Nurse, 2*(3), 9–13.

Hartshorn, J.C. (1988). The power to influence. *Heart & Lung, 17*(1), 27A–28A, 30A.

Holle, M.L., & Blatchley, M.E. (1987). *Introduction to leadership and management in nursing* (2nd ed.). Boston: Jones and Bartlett.

Johnson, M.J., & Wroblewski, M. (1989). Litigation stress in nurses. *Nursing Management, 20*(10), 23–25.

Johnson, P.T. (1988). Critical care visitation: An ethical dilemma. *Critical Care Nurse, 8*(6), 72,75–78.

Kohler, P. (1988). Model of shared control. *Journal of Gerontological Nursing, 14*(7), 21–25,

Martin, D.A., & Redland, A.R. (1988). Legal and ethical issues in resuscitation and withholding of treatment. *Critical Care Nursing Quarterly, 10*(4), 1–8.

McFayden, J.A. (1989). Who will speak for me? *Nursing Times, 85*(6), 45–48.

McMullen, P. (1988). Advocacy can save you from litigation. *Nursing Connections, 1*(4), 54–56.

Mitchell, C. (1987). Steadying the hand that feeds. *American Journal of Nursing, 87,* 293–294, 296.

O'Mara, R.J. (1987). Ethical dilemmas with advance directives: Living wills and do not resuscitate orders. *Critical Care Nursing Quarterly, 10*(2), 17–28.

Pagana, K.D. (1987). Let's stop calling ourselves "Patient Advocates." *Nursing 87, 17*(2), 51.

Phillips, L.R. (1987). Respect basic human rights. *Journal of Gerontological Nursing, 13*(3), 36–39.

Reedy, N.J., Minoque, J.P., & Sterk, M.B. (1987). The critically ill neonate: Dilemmas in perinatal ethics. *Critical Care Nursing Quarterly, 10*(2), 56–64.

Robinson, M.B. 91985). Patient advocacy and the nurse: Is there a conflict of interest? *Nursing Forum, 22,* 58–63.

Selby, T.L. (1988). Nurses excel as advocates for patients. *American Nurse, 20*(2), 1, 7–8.

Silver, M. (1987). Using restraint. *American Journal of Nursing, 87,* 1414–1415.

Tappen, R.M. (1989). *Nursing leadership and management: Concepts and practice* (2nd ed.). Philadelphia: Davis.

Thompson, J., Pender, K.K., & Hoffman-Schmitt, J. (1987). Retaining rights of impaired elderly. *Journal of Gerontological Nursing, 13*(3), 20–25.

Yorker, B. (1988). The nurses' use of restraint with a neurologically impaired patient. *Journal of Neuroscience Nursing, 20,* 390–392.

Understanding and Using Research Findings

Objectives

After completing this chapter, you should be able to:

1. *Demonstrate a beginning understanding of research terminology.*
2. *Identify the steps in the research process.*
3. *Cite basic differences in quantitative and qualitative approaches to nursing research.*
4. *Describe the Nuremberg Code for safeguarding research subjects.*
5. *Use a framework for understanding research reports and identifying how research findings can be implemented in the clinical setting.*

What if you as a staff nurse had a tool that could help you identify which of several diabetic teaching methods was most effective for your patients? Or what if you could determine which of the clean-catch specimen containers was easiest for staff nurses to use correctly? Or suppose you could demonstrate to your head nurse that decreasing shift rotation on a particular unit would actually be more effective? Would this not be a marvelous tool?

The process that could help you do these kinds of things is nursing research. *Research* is a form of systematic inquiry for purposes of decision making, problem solving, or prediction based upon orderly scientific methods (Polit & Hungler, 1988). Like management, research is often another area that beginning nurses sometimes feel is not directly related to their patient care practice. In reality, all nurses need research skills and knowledge if they are to practice safely and effectively. Without it, nursing decisions may be made based on invalid assumptions, unexamined customs, or costly trial-and-error experience.

If this is true, why is it that we do not see nursing research practiced more frequently? Why do staff nurses sometimes feel that research has little value for them in the practice setting? One reason is that nurses traditionally have not been taught to read research reports and have not been assisted to apply these findings in their clinical practice. All too frequently they are left out of the formal research process. By becoming more knowledgeable about research, learning to identify clinical problems that can be addressed by research, and applying research findings in practice, nurses can gain the benefits of this process and can, in addition, contribute to the development of nursing knowledge.

In this chapter you will learn about the scientific method and the research process. Terminology important to reading and understanding research reports will be presented. Two basic types of research will be presented, with examples of each. Participating in ongoing research will be discussed, along with legal and ethical considerations in dealing with patients during the research process. Finally, ways will be discussed in which you as a student can begin to understand research better.

THE SCIENTIFIC METHOD AND THE RESEARCH PROCESS

Understanding research begins with an understanding of the scientific method and the research process. Like the nursing process, the scientific method involves specific steps that assist the researcher in setting out the problem to be examined and the means to solve the problem. The scientific method consists of the following steps:

1. Identifying the problem
2. Collecting information

3. Making a hypothesis
4. Designing the experiment
5. Testing the hypothesis
6. Generalizing
7. Testing the generalization.

As you will have noticed, the scientific method has much in common with the nursing process. Both identify an area of concern to be examined and begin the process of gathering information (assessment). Then the scientist develops a hypothesis of what is actually occurring (diagnosis). To test this hypothesis, the scientist plans certain actions that he or she expects to produce certain results, which he or she then evaluates in the light of his hypothesis (planning, intervention, and evaluation). The process begins over again as the results are generalized and more experiments are planned to confirm the validity of the generalizations.

Like nursing process and the scientific method, the research process itself has discrete steps that may vary according to the type of research done. The typical research study might have the following steps:

- Statement of the problem
- Review of the literature
- Development of theoretical framework
- Identification of variables
- Formation of hypotheses
- Selection of research design
- Collection of data
- Analysis of data
- Presentation of findings
- Interpretation of findings.

These steps will be discussed in more detail in the section dealing with understanding research reports. As in the nursing process, establishing a formal sequence of steps assists the nurse in addressing the problem in an orderly way. This same pattern can later be followed by other researchers who may also be interested in the topic.

As a new graduate, you might find yourself involved in research in a number of ways. First, patients you are assigned to care for may be involved as subjects in a research study. You must be knowledgeable about the study and the research process so that you can plan your care so as not to compromise the study. Second, you may be able to see situations where research might help answer nursing questions and to suggest them as possible topics to your head nurse or clinical specialist. Finally, as you participate in continuing education and in inservice presentations and as you read nursing journals, you may identify knowledge gained through research that will allow you to make positive changes in your nursing practice.

UNDERSTANDING RESEARCH TERMINOLOGY AND PROCESS

One reason nurses fail to use research findings is that it is often difficult to understand what the findings mean unless the nurse has a basic understanding of research language. This does not mean that the nurse must be a statistician or a doctorally prepared nurse researcher in order to use research information, but it does mean that all nurses should have a basic understanding of research terminology and the research process.

Research Terminology

You should be familiar with a number of terms routinely used by nurse researchers. These will be discussed individually, and then the following example will be used to illustrate their use.

A group of nurse researchers was interested in learning if a nurse's own experience with pain could influence her assessment of a patient's

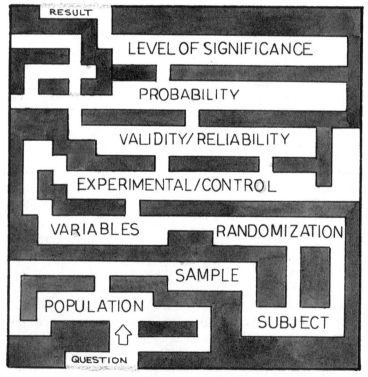

Understanding the terminology used in research will help you to move more easily through what may seem a confusing maze.

pain (Holm et al., 1989) They wondered if this experience might bias the nurses' assessment of patients in pain. To answer this question, they first began by reviewing studies done by other nurses to see what was known about this phenomenon. Then they designed their own study. Using three questionnaires, they asked 134 nurses about their own experiences with pain and their perception of patient pain. The results of the study indicated that nurses who had experienced pain tended to evaluate their patient's pain as being more severe than did nurses who had not personally experienced pain.

To evaluate whether this difference was significant, the researchers used a statistical test to determine whether the differences in the two groups of nurses could be simply a matter of chance. In this case, the difference was significant, and the researchers concluded that a nurse's previous experience with pain might be associated with a higher assessment of patient pain.

In this example, the population that the nurse researchers wanted to know more about included nurses who had mild to severe personal experiences with pain. In a research study, the *population* is that entire group of individuals about whom you seek information. Generally, it is not possible to obtain information about an entire population, so researchers select a representative group to examine; they make inferences about the population based upon this *sample*. The degree to which the sample, or selected group, can provide information about the population from which it is drawn depends on how like, or how representative, the sample is of the population. Each member of the sample is called a *subject*.

Obviously, the way in which each subject is chosen is very important. Researchers generally like to assign subjects to comparison groups by the process of *randomization*. This ensures that each subject has an equal opportunity of being chosen for any particular group and that any differences between the groups are due to chance. Frequently, it is impossible to assign subjects randomly to groups, and another method of sorting is utilized, as was done in our example.

The term *variable* is used to describe something in the environment that varies, or changes. In our example, the variables of interest included previous experience with pain, assessment of patient pain, and various sociodemographic variables such as age, sex, and ethnicity. *Independent variables* are those variables that vary by themselves, or that can be caused to vary. In our example, the independent variable is whether the nurse had had previous experience with pain. The *dependent variable* is that which changes as a result of the independent variable. In our example, the dependent variable is assessment of patient pain, which was affected by whether the nurse had personal experience with pain. Other variables are known as *extraneous variables*. These are variables that might also affect the dependent variable and could confuse the relationship between the independent and dependent variables. In our example, extraneous variables might have included such things as experience with a family member's pain or recent attendance at a workshop that emphasized the underassessment of patient pain.

The terms *experimental* and *control* are used to refer to groups of subjects in a research design. Having two groups allows the researcher to make comparisons and to evaluate the effect of the independent variable (*e.g.*, a treatment) on the dependent variable. One group, the experimental group, can be exposed to the treatment while the other, the control group, is not. The function of the control group is to help the researcher determine that the change in the experimental group is due to the treatment.

Many nursing studies cannot be carried out in the classical experimental way because patients cannot be subjected to harmful treatments and helpful treatments cannot be withheld. In our example the researchers did not use control and experimental groups in the traditional sense. Instead they formed the comparison groups on the basis of self-reported pain experiences and provided information to show that the groups are otherwise similar.

The terms *validity* and *reliability* refer to the degree to which the research data reflect the phenomenon investigated accurately. *Validity* is defined as the degree to which an assessment tool actually measures what it is supposed to measure. In our example, it was important that the questionnaire used to measure perception of patient pain actually did so.

Reliability is defined as the degree of consistency or dependability with which an assessment tool measures something. If an assessment tool is reliable, it will produce the same results when used again, or in different circumstances. If the questionnaire used to evaluate perception of patient pain was only reliable when the nurse had an hour to assess the patient, it would not be accurate in other, more common circumstances of patient assessment.

Probability refers to the likelihood of something happening. In research reports we are interested in the likelihood of a result being the result of chance variation rather than a result of the interaction of the dependent and independent variables. Through the use of statistical techniques the researcher can identify the probability of the observed result being due to chance variation. This is generally stated in the form of a mathematical expression, for example, $p < 0.05$, meaning that there is less than a 5 percent probability that this result could be explained by chance.

Another term associated with probability is the *level of significance*. This is a figure, chosen by the researcher, that identifies the level of probability that will be judged to be significant. Frequently used levels of significance are 0.05 and 0.01, with the latter being a more conservative level, in that only one time in 100 events of this type could the result be expected to be due to chance rather than to the interaction of the dependent and independent variables.

Readers of research reports will also find references to statistical tests. Statistical tests are used to determine whether the results are, in fact, significant at the level identified by the researcher. Each statistical test has a different purpose and can be used only when specific criteria are met. In the research report, the researcher generally gives both a figure for the test and one for the level of probability. This allows the researcher to make judgments about the hypotheses.

It is important to understand that there is a difference between statistical significance and clinical significance. A result can be statistically significant without producing clinically important changes. In a study of bladder decompression described in the following section, nurses found that there were statistically significant changes in blood pressure and heart rate in patients whose bladders were emptied by stages when compared with patients whose bladders were emptied at one time. However, these changes had little clinical significance, because they did not indicate any important physiological change in the patients' status.

Beginning readers of research reports who have not yet had coursework in statistics can still understand the implications of the research findings by reading the researchers' interpretation of findings. Here the various statistical tests are interpreted and the hypotheses are either rejected or not rejected.

There are additional figures reported in most research reports that are easier for the beginning reader of research to understand. These include the mean, or average score of subjects on the variables examined; the range of scores from highest to lowest; and the standard deviation (SD). In our example, the mean age of the nurses in the study was 31.6 years. The range was from 21 to 61 years. The researchers also provide information on how much variation from the average age was observed. This measure is called the SD. A high SD would mean that in the sample a large number of nurses were considerably older and younger than the average age. A small SD would mean that more nurses were closer in age to the average. This is important information for readers of research reports. If the group to whom you wish to apply the research findings is not similar to the group studied, the results may be quite different. Information on the mean, range, and SD helps readers to make judgments about the applicability of the results to their own settings.

The Research Process

Earlier we listed the steps in the research process. It is helpful for the reader of research to understand what is done in each step of the process and why it is important to follow them. The first step in the process is the

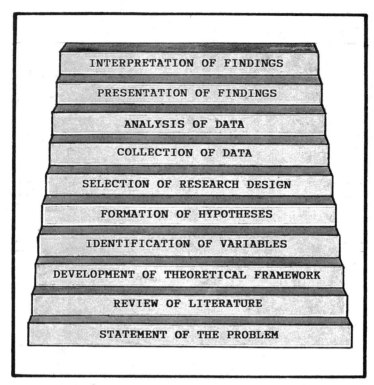

INTERPRETATION OF FINDINGS

PRESENTATION OF FINDINGS

ANALYSIS OF DATA

COLLECTION OF DATA

SELECTION OF RESEARCH DESIGN

FORMATION OF HYPOTHESES

IDENTIFICATION OF VARIABLES

DEVELOPMENT OF THEORETICAL FRAMEWORK

REVIEW OF LITERATURE

STATEMENT OF THE PROBLEM

Researchers follow a series of well-defined steps that help them to approach the question in a systematic manner.

identification, or *statement of the problem*. This might seem to you to be self-evident: What you want to know *is* the statement of the problem. Frequently, however, what we want to know is too generalized to be properly researched and the first task of the researcher is to define and circumscribe the problem carefully. In our example, perhaps the nurse researchers had initially felt that nurses who had experienced pain themselves might be more sympathetic to patients in pain and that such nurses would consequently evaluate patients' degree of pain differently from nurses who had not experienced pain. This might be stated as, "Personal experience can influence perception." At this point the "problem" is not stated clearly enough to design a study to investigate it. The researchers must isolate the specific thing to be observed (dependent variable); the specific things thought to cause, predict, or be associated with it (independent variables); and the nature of the relationship between them. In our example, the statement of the problem might have been phrased, "Is assessment of patient pain significantly influenced by the intensity of the nurse's personal experience with pain?"

The second step in the research process is the *review of the literature*. Again, this is a step that beginning researchers often feel is less important than getting to the task at hand. However, becoming familiar with what is already known about the problem, including what other investigations have been done and what populations have been studied, can save the researcher much time and effort. Another important reason for reviewing what has been done is so that the planned research can be constructed in an orderly way to add to the development of nursing knowledge. It is the responsibility of all nurse researchers to relate their investigations to the established body of nursing knowledge and to the work being done by other researchers.

The third step assists the researcher further to relate this specific study to established knowledge. This *development of the theoretical framework* requires the researcher to set the stage for this particular project. It defines the way in which the researcher views nursing and the particular problem to be investigated. In research reports the reader will often find a discussion of a particular nursing theory and how this relates to the planned research. This linking of research to theory helps to connect the various investigations into a fabric that can help us to understand better not only the problem currently studied, but the larger realm of nursing as well.

The third, fourth, and fifth steps in the research process involve *identification of variables, formation of hypotheses,* and *selection of research design*. This is when the methods of the study are defined. The first step involves teasing out the specific dependent variable to be studied, which in our example you know to be assessment of the level of the patient's pain. Often it is hard to identify the specific elements that might be causing the change in the dependent variable. Nursing is a complex activity, and it is challenging to identify the most important variables without eliminating others that might significantly influence the variable of interest. In our example, you know that the most important independent variable examined was the nurses' previous experience with pain. Other variables examined included age, sex, and ethnicity.

Once the variables have been ascertained, the researcher must identify the nature of the association between or among them and state a hypothesis. A hypothesis is a statement of predicted relationships between the variables. In our example the hypothesis might have been phrased as, "Mean level of assessed pain in patients differs for different levels of previous pain experience in nurses." You can see that the hypothesis frequently is a restatement of the problem.

There is another way in which hypotheses can be stated that frequently is confusing to beginning readers of research reports. This form of hypothesis is called the *null hypothesis*. It is used for statistical clarity when the researcher hopes to disprove an assumption. If the hypothesis in our example had been stated in the null form, it might have read, "There will be no difference in the mean level of assessed patient pain based on level of previous exposure to pain in nurses." It is important to understand that the researcher actually does expect to see a relationship and that the negative form is used to be able to reject the hypothesis.

The selection of the research design is actually determined by the nature of the variables and the type of relationship thought to exist between them. The research design must be appropriate to the study planned; otherwise the conclusions drawn will be invalid. Many nurse researchers work collaboratively with statisticians at this point to ensure that the planned research design and analysis of data will provide the type of information the researcher is seeking.

Once the variables are identified, the hypotheses are stated, and the research design is decided, the researcher implements the study and goes ahead with *collection of data.* In our example, the researchers administered the questionnaires and gathered data on all three variables: the nurses' previous experience with pain; sociodemographic variables, including age, sex, and ethnicity; and the assessed level of patient pain. The next step in the process is the *analysis of data;* during this process the specific statistical tests appropriate for the study are performed. The researchers summarize information about the subjects studied and give the results of their statistical tests.

The last two steps in the research process are the *presentation of findings* and *interpretation of findings.* Often they are presented together in the research report. The presentation of findings involves reporting the data gathered. As you have seen, this generally includes giving information on the sociodemographic variables as well as the dependent and other independent variables. Usually, the data are reported in terms of mean score, range, and SD. Following this, the results of the analysis are presented and the hypothesis is either rejected or not rejected. The importance of the findings is discussed, including the implications of the results for nursing practice. This is an important section for readers of research reports. Although it may be difficult to understand the intricacies of the statistical analysis completely, it is generally very clear what the researchers feel are the implications for nursing practice. They will make recommendations to practicing nurses and to other nurse researchers who may want to repeat the study or to investigate other questions suggested by the research.

An important part of the research process involves the dissemination of findings to other nurses. This is frequently done by publishing research reports or by presenting research at nursing conferences. The beginning reader of research reports will find an increased understanding of reported research by becoming involved in research conferences and in nursing research discussion groups and by regularly reading nursing research journals.

TYPES OF RESEARCH

As mentioned earlier, not all types of problems can be addressed in the same way, and the design of the research must fit the type of problem being studied. The two major types of research are called quantitative and qualitative.

Quantitative Research

Quantitative research emphasizes experimentation and statistical analysis. It is generally what is thought of when research is mentioned. Generally, quantitative research focuses on measurable observation and is very objective and tries to be value-free. The three principal types of quantitative research are experimental, quasi-experimental, and nonexperimental designs.

The experimental research design, for example, has three characteristics: (1) Subjects are randomly assigned to groups; (2) the researcher

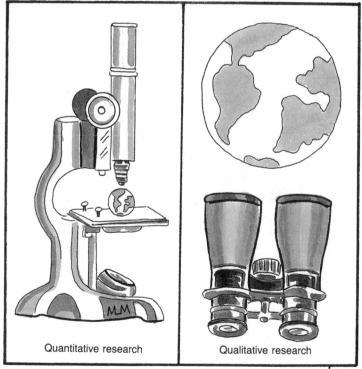

| Quantitative research | Qualitative research |

Quantitative and qualitative research look at the world from a different viewpoint.

manipulates (gives a treatment to) one group; and (3) the other group, called the control group, does not receive the treatment and is used for comparison purposes. This structure allows the researcher to observe differences between the two groups and to make conclusions about the effect of the treatment from empirical observations.

Qualitative Research

Qualitative research aims at a different sort of information. Unlike quantitative research, it is concerned with the subjective and contextual; that is, it looks at phenomena of interest in their environment, rather than attempting to isolate them, as is frequently done in quantitative research. Examples of qualitative research methodologies include phenomenology and ethnography.

The aim of *phenomenology*, for example, is "to describe experience as it is lived by people" (Munhall & Oiler, 1986, p 70). The information sought draws upon the patient's subjective interpretation of an experience, which itself reflects previous experiences as well as current factors. A phenomenological approach was used by Riemen (1986) in her examination of how patients perceived their nurses as caring or noncaring. Other examples of research that might use a phenomenological approach include the examination of what it means to experience pain, the approach of death, or recovery from disease.

Ethnography is probably best known as a tool of anthropologists who seek to describe the characteristics of a particular culture. The culture can be very large and inclusive, such as the health culture of the Hmong refugees, or very small, such as the health practices of a single family. The ethnographic researcher becomes involved in the culture being studied and tries to describe it as completely as possible. Rather than trying to isolate variables, as the quantitative researcher would do, the ethnographer tries to include as many as possible. As the ethnographer gathers information, themes and patterns become evident, and the researcher gains an understanding of "norms, values, belief systems, language, rituals, economics and role behaviors" in the group studied (Munhall & Oiler, 1986, p. 148).

Combined Research Strategies

Both quantitative and qualitative research are important for nursing. Sometimes a quantitative research design is the most effective; other times qualitative approaches are most appropriate. Many researchers are now combining both approaches; this is called *triangulation research*. This allows researchers to look at the phenomena being studied from two different perspectives that can add depth and validity to the study.

To compare the approaches, consider the following decision that staff nurses on a surgical unit might want to make. Suppose they are considering a variety of brochures designed to help prepare patients and their families for surgery. The brochures vary in terms of the amount of detail provided, the variety of illustrations, and the degree to which they involve nurses in the teaching process. The staff members identify two brochures that look promising and attempt to compare them.

A quantitative research design would allow the nurses to compare the effectiveness of the brochures in a number of ways. They could identify two groups of patients that were basically similar and have each group read one of the brochures. The nurses could assess individuals for physiological signs and symptoms of nervousness such as respiratory and heart rate before and after reading the brochures. They could assess understanding by giving individuals an objective pre-test and post-test. These quantitative measures would allow them to compare the results of using the two brochures and could help them make a decision on which best reduced physiological signs of anxiety and increased understanding.

A qualitative research design might approach the question of which brochure was better by asking the patients about the feelings they had before they had read the brochures and how they were different afterward. It might ask such questions as, "What concerns did you have about the surgery before reading the brochure?" "Did you feel more at ease about the surgery after reading it?" "Do you still have questions or concerns that we can answer?" The answers from patients who had read one brochure could be compared with those who had read another, and judgments could be made about which one was most effective.

The advantages of a quantitative design are that it is easy to measure differences and to understand their significance. In the first example, the staff nurses could actually measure the difference in their patients' physiological responses and the difference in their scores on pretests and posttests. Using one type of brochure with one group of patients and the second brochure with another, similar group of patients, they could then compare the numerical differences using a statistical measure to determine whether the differences were actually significant. The disadvantage is that this may not actually tell them much about how the patients felt about their impending surgeries and how the brochures might have influenced these feelings.

The advantage of a qualitative measure is that it allows you to address the question more broadly, using as a primary source of information the patient's subjective response. The disadvantage is that it is harder to compare the responses of the different patients.

As mentioned, nurses are finding that a combination approach using both quantitative and qualitative methods is helpful. Because the problems nurses are interested in are not generally ones that can be isolated and examined in a laboratory setting, where all the variables can be controlled, and because it is usually not possible to use a traditional experimental approach to see which interventions are most effective, the use of a combined strategy that includes a qualitative as well as a quantitative approach is often most informative.

LEGAL AND ETHICAL CONSIDERATIONS

Regardless of the type of research done, the researcher must be concerned with certain considerations. The first has to with consent.

Before any research project can be initiated, the individuals who will be the subjects in the study must be informed about the study and give their consent to participate. It is important to recognize that just as nurses have an important duty to serve as patient advocates in the daily delivery of nursing care, they also have an obligation to see that patients are safeguarded during any research study. Certain types of patients require particular protection, such as the very young and the mentally incompetent.

LoBiondo-Wood and Haber (1986) point out that the first codification of principles to govern research upon human subjects was developed during the Nuremberg Tribunal. The code was a response to the appalling experimentation conducted by German researchers upon prisoners during the World War II. To safeguard patients' ethical and legal rights, the following rules for ethical research were developed:

1. Voluntary consent of the human subject is essential.
2. Experiments should be so designed and based on the results of animal experimentation and knowledge of the natural history of the disease or other problems that the anticipated results will justify the experiment.
3. The degree of risk to be taken by the subject should never exceed the potential humanitarian importance of the problem to be studied.
4. Through all stages of the experiment the highest degree of skill and care should be required of those who conduct or engage in it, and the experiment should be conducted only by scientifically qualified persons.
5. At any time during the course of the experiment, the human subject should be at liberty to end participation in the experiment.
6. The scientist in charge must be prepared to terminate the experiment at any stage if there is probable cause to believe that continuation of the experiment is likely to result in injury, disability, or the death of the subject (p. 31).

Just as patients must give informed consent for any medical procedure, they must be fully informed about any proposed research before they can legally give their consent. The formal consent form generally describes the purposes of the research, the procedures that will be followed, the risks, discomforts, and benefits expected. The subject is generally guaranteed anonymity or at least confidentiality. If alternative treatments are available, this must also be described. Finally, the subject is assured that participation is voluntary and can be terminated at any time.

Similarly, just as it is appropriate for a staff nurse to inform a physician of patient questions that indicate a lack of understanding of a planned procedure, so is it appropriate for the staff nurse to communicate to the nurse researcher any misgivings or misunderstandings a subject may voice concerning proposed research participation.

Generally, research that is undertaken in a health care setting requires approval by one or more review boards. There may be an institutional review board that evaluates and approves all proposals before they can be implemented. If the research is being conducted in conjunction with a school of nursing, medicine, or other academic discipline, that institution will also have a review committee that will evaluate and approve the research proposal. Granting agencies may have yet another approval process. The aim of these multiple reviews is to ensure that the legal and ethical rights of patients as research subjects are protected.

PARTICIPATING IN RESEARCH

We have already mentioned one important way in which staff nurses can assist the research process by helping to ensure that patient rights, both ethical and legal, are safeguarded. Others include helping to identify nursing problems that need research, assisting with ongoing research, and helping to implement the results of nursing research in the practice setting.

Identifying Problems for Research

Staff nurses are in an ideal position to identify important research needs. First, nurses generally are excellent observers, because they have been carefully trained in the assessment skills so important to the research process. Second, nurses are the ones responsible for putting the whole complex of patient care together; as a consequence, it is they who notice when the overall plan of care is ineffective.

Typically, a topic for research might suggest itself in the form of a problem or a question. For example, one group of nurses wondered whether it was really necessary, as some nursing texts and articles have suggested, to empty a patient's distended bladder in stages, rather than all at once. The argument for clamping a catheter for a period of time once

1000 ml has been drained implies that sudden decompression can result in syncope, sepsis, hemorrhage, and shock (Bristoll et al., 1989). The nurse researchers designed a study to test whether there was any difference in patient response to complete bladder emptying and staged emptying. The importance of finding the answer to this question included the fact that if complete emptying was safe, both nursing time and patient discomfort could be minimized.

Following appropriate research protocols, the nurses obtained written consent from six patients as they were referred for urinary catheterization to relieve distention. The six were randomly assigned to two groups: one to have complete bladder emptying and the second to have staged bladder emptying. This random assignment helped to ensure that the patient groups were likely to be similar.

Baseline and subsequent measures of blood pressure, heart rate, and presence of blood in urine were monitored in the two groups. Each sample was cultured for presence of bacteria. A comparison of the data from the two groups showed that although there were differences in the two groups as reflected in blood pressure and heart rate changes, these differences were not clinically significant. Patients who experienced complete bladder emptying did just as well as those who were treated in the conservative manner.

The nurse researchers invited others to replicate their study and suggested that complete bladder emptying appeared to be more comfortable and as safe as staged bladder emptying.

Other routinely implemented nursing measures need to be critically evaluated. Staff nurses are in a position to identify these questionable areas and to suggest studies that can explore them.

Assisting with Ongoing Research

Whether a nurse decides to be actively involved in research, it is likely at some point that the patients under his or her care will be. It is important for staff nurses to understand the types of things that can affect research results and to help ensure that the data collected will be as accurate as possible. The following situations can pose a threat to the reliability and validity of a research study.

One factor that can pose a threat to reliability and validity is measurement error. If the nurses investigating the question of complete bladder drainage had not taken care to measure the variables of blood pressure, pulse, and presence of blood and bacteria in the urine carefully, the results of their study could have been misleading. Measurement errors can occur for a number of reasons. The person taking the reading may fail to follow the protocols established for the study. The environment itself, such as the temperature or humidity level, may affect the variables measured. The reagent strips used to test for presence of blood may be difficult to read. All these factors can affect the results obtained. Nurses involved in caring for patients who are involved in research studies can help to identify those threats to measurement that might result in misleading or inaccurate data. By drawing these to the attention of the researcher, it may be possible to correct or control for such factors and to safeguard the integrity of the research.

In addition to measurement error, a number of other factors can threaten the research study. These are called subject variables; they include history, maturation, testing, selection, and mortality.

History refers to the fact that events other than the experimental variable can affect outcome. Suppose, for example, that researchers were studying a technique to reduce anxiety in preoperative patients and that during the time of the study there was a fire drill in the hospital. The noise and commotion of the fire drill might strongly affect the level of anxiety patients experienced. This could then make it difficult for the researchers to evaluate the effect of a treatment designed to reduce anxiety.

Maturation refers to the fact that subjects are growing and changing and that differences measured from one point in time to another may be due to changes in maturation. This is especially important in research studies that deal with populations undergoing rapid changes, such as the patients in a pediatric unit.

Testing refers to the fact that a testing procedure can itself pose a threat to research integrity, because it can produce changes in a patient. This is particularly true if the research design uses a time-series format. If the experience of being tested makes it easier for a patient to respond to the question a second, third, or fourth time, the changes may be due to experience with the test instrument rather than to the nursing intervention the test is designed to measure.

Selection refers to the sorting of subjects into control and experimental groups. If the assignment to groups is not random, as would be true of patients who volunteer to participate in a control or experimental group, there may be significant undetected differences between the two groups. In the bladder catheterization study, for example, if patients had been allowed to choose which group they would be placed in rather than being randomly assigned, this might have affected the outcome of the study. Suppose some of the patients had previously been catheterized with full bladders and were comfortable with the procedure. Suppose they all volunteered to be a part of the complete bladder decompression group. These patients might have been basically different from patients in the other group, who might have been more likely to be anxious and to have higher blood pressures and heart rates. These basic, undetected differences between groups could have produced misleading results.

Mortality refers to the loss of subjects from a study. Another name for this phenomenon is *attrition*. Even when the two groups being compared are basically similar, the differential loss of group members may change the composition of the groups. This is an even greater problem when the groups may not be basically equivalent. If, in the study of the preoperative brochure, a considerable number of patients in the other hospital surgical unit failed to complete the questionnaires and if the ones who failed to do so were all unable to read the questionnaire because it was too difficult for them, the researchers could make faulty conclusions about the effectiveness of the brochure in that group of patients. The fact that these patients were lost to the study could result in the researchers drawing incorrect conclusions from their data.

The staff nurse is in a good position to help observe for these threats to the research study. By helping to ensure that other variables do not affect the outcome, the results obtained and the interpretations made will be as reliable and valid as possible.

Implementing Research Findings

Staff nurses who read research reports and who look for opportunities to apply these findings in practice can make an important contribution not only to patient care but also to the expansion of nursing knowledge. Implementing findings involves identifying research that can be helpful in an individual nursing environment, working collaboratively to introduce changes based on the research report, and evaluating the effectiveness of the changes. This should sound to you like the nursing process taken one step further, and in fact it is. The nurse who reads research journals and assesses reports for application, say, to the care of orthopedic patients, may find that other nurses in orthopedic units report what looks like a very effective way to prepare patients for total joint replacement surgery. The nurse might then bring in the research report for his or her colleagues and supervisor to read. They might then get assistance from the clinical nurse specialist, the nurse researcher, and/or the nurse administrator to test the effectiveness of the preoperative preparation in their orthopedic unit.

The research design would be chosen and a decision would be made about which patients would participate as subjects. The plan would be reviewed by the institution's research committee. Consents and protocols providing for the patients' legal and ethical protection would be developed and the data would be carefully and accurately gathered. The nurses would then be able to make judgments about the effectiveness of the preoperative preparation based upon their research. This would allow them to institute changes in their own unit that would benefit their orthopedic patients and families and would allow them to share these findings with other nurses by writing a report of their replication for publication.

READING RESEARCH REPORTS: A GUIDE

As a student, perhaps the best way for you to become more familiar with the research process and more knowledgeable about current research is to read and then begin to use information from published research reports.

To begin, identify an area of nursing that is of interest to you. This could be a clinical area, such as geriatrics or obstetrics, or could reflect a concern such as the nurse's role in organ donation.

Go to the nursing literature and find what has been written about the problem. Sources of information about what research exists in a particular area include the *Cumulative Index to Nursing and Allied Health,* the *Index Medicus,* and computer databases such as Medline and Dialogue. These contain bibliographic information on articles published in many journals and can provide a starting place for you to discover the state of nursing knowledge in the area of interest. Your reference librarian can help you locate the various indexes and provide information and assistance with computer searches.

Once you have located several titles of interest, consult the listing of periodicals for your library. If the library you are using does not have those particular journals, the reference librarian may be able to suggest other libraries that carry them or help you to obtain them through an interlibrary loan agreement.

Generally, it is helpful, once you have obtained the research articles, to make copies of them for your own use so that you are free to make notations as questions or concerns occur to you. As you read the articles, use the study guide on pages 308–309 to assess the usefulness of the research report for your own practice.

SUMMARY

In this chapter we have reviewed the research process and compared it to the scientific method. We have discussed research terminology that is necessary for beginning users of research data to understand, including such concepts as population, sample, subject, selection, randomization, variable, control, experimental, validity, reliability, probability, and significance. We have identified two basic types of research, quantitative and

(*Text continues on page 310*)

Reading Research Reports

Author:
Title:
Journal name and issue:

Statement of the Problem: What were the researchers attempting to learn about? Is it clear to you what they were investigating? What questions would you like to ask them if you could?

Review of the Literature: What do the researchers tell you about the level of our knowledge regarding this problem? Are there are research reports that you might want to review? Does this research seem to address the questions earlier research has raised?

Theoretical Framework: Do the researchers indicate how their study fits into nursing knowledge as a whole? Do they relate their study to theories from other fields, such as education, psychology, or sociology?

Identification of Variables: Do the researchers clearly point out dependent and independent variables? Do the researchers explain how the variables will be measured?

Formation of Hypotheses: Do the researchers clearly indicate how the dependent and independent variables are linked? Is it clear what their research is designed to test or to examine?

Continued

Reading Research Reports (Continued)

Research Design: Do the researchers say what type of design they have chosen? Can you see things that might interfere with their data collection? Have the researchers taken these threats into account and attempted to control for them?

Collection of Data: How did the researchers go about obtaining their information? Did they provide for voluntary consent and withdrawal of subjects at any point desired?

Analysis of Data: Do the researchers tell you how they analyzed the data? If this is a quantitative study, do they identify the statistical tests used and the level of significance they have chosen? If a qualitative approach is used, do the researchers describe what techniques have been used to draw their conclusions?

Presentation and Interpretation of Findings: Based upon their analysis, what do the researchers say about the hypotheses? Do they present their findings objectively? Do they relate their findings to earlier research and their theoretical framework? Do they indicate how their findings can be used in practice? How will this information help you in your clinical practice? What additional questions does it raise?

Your Contribution: With the information from this research report, what changes might you want to make in your own practice? What implications does this have for you as a student? With whom would you need to share this information? What are the implications of not using the knowledge you have gained from this research report?

qualitative, and discussed differences between them, providing examples of each.

We have discussed the stages of the research process and what the responsibilities of the researcher are at each point in the process. The specific legal and ethical responsibilities of researchers to protect the rights of subjects were presented. Responsibilities of nurses involved in caring for patients who are subjects in a research study were discussed, including the need to be aware of threats to the integrity of the study, such as measurement errors and the subject variables referred to as history, maturation, testing, selection, and mortality. Finally, a framework for beginning to read and integrate information from research reports has been provided.

Unless the results of nursing research find their way into the clinical practice of nurses at the bedside, it will continue to be less than fully effective. Nurses providing direct care can assist in validating research findings and in suggesting other areas for investigation, and they can help to ensure that ongoing research is conducted under optimal circumstances. Nursing research is a tool that nurses functioning at all levels can use effectively to improve the care of patients.

Study Questions/Activities

1. What are the eight steps in the research process?
2. How do quantitative and qualitative approaches to research vary?
3. What is meant by the terms *population, sample, subject, selection, randomization, variable control, experimental, validity, reliability, probability,* and *significance?*
4. Why is it important for nurse researchers to include a review of literature and theoretical framework?
5. What are the provisions of the Nuremberg Code?
6. How can beginning nurses participate in the research process?
7. What area of nursing of interest to you might you begin to explore through nursing research reports?
8. Choose and review one nursing research article using the format suggested.

REFERENCES

Bristoll, S.L., Fadden, T., Fehring, R.J., Rohde, L., Smith, P.K, & Wohlitz, B.A. (1989). The mythical danger of rapid urinary drainage. *American Journal of Nursing, 89*(3), 344–345.

Holm, K., Cohen, F., Dudas, S., Medema, P.G, & Allen, B.L. (1989). Effect of personal pain experience on pain assessment. *Image, 21*(2), 72–75.

LoBiondo-Wood, G., & Haber, J. (1986). *Nursing research: Critical appraisal and utilization.* St. Louis: C.V. Mosby.

Munhall, P., & Oiler, C. (1986). *Nursing research: A qualitative perspective.* Norwalk, Conn.: Appleton-Century-Crofts.

Polit, D., & Hungler, B. (1988). *Nursing research: Principles and methods.* Philadelphia: J.B. Lippincott.

Riemen, D.J (1986). The essential structure of a caring interaction: Doing phenomenology. In Munhall, P., & Oiler, C. *Nursing research: A qualitative perspective.* Norwalk, Conn.: Appleton-Century-Crofts.

SUGGESTIONS FOR FURTHER READING

Chinn, P.L. (1986). *Nursing research methodology: Issues and implementation.* Rockville, Md.: Aspen Publishers.

Polit, D., & Hungler, P. (1988). *Essentials of nursing research.* Philadelphia: J.B. Lippincott.

Porter, E.J. (1989). The qualitative-quantitative dualism. *Image, 2(12),* 98–102.

Index

Page numbers followed by f indicate figures; those followed by t indicate tabular material.